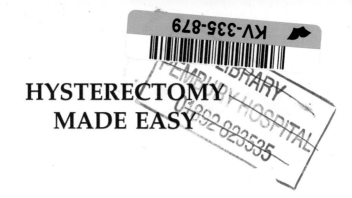

HYSTERECTOMY MADE EASY

System requirement:
- Windows XP or above
- Power DVD player (Software)
- Windows media player 10.0 version or above (Software)

Accompanying CD ROM is playable only in Computer and not in CD player.

Kindly wait for few seconds for CD to autorun. If it does not autorun then please follow the steps:
- Click on my computer
- Click the CD drive labelled JAYPEE and after opening the Drive, kindly double click the file Jaypee

CD CONTENTS

A080251

WP 468

Published by

Jitendar P Vij
Jaypee Brothers Medical Publishers (P) Ltd
B-3, EMCA House, 23/23B Ansari Road, Daryaganj, **New Delhi** 110 002, India
Phones: +91-11-23272143, +91-11-23272703, +91-11-23282021, +91-11-23245672
Rel: 32558559   Fax: +91-11-23276490, +91-11-23245683
e-mail: jaypee@jaypeebrothers.com   Visit our website: www.jaypeebrothers.com

Branches

- 2/B, Akruti Society, Jodhpur Gam Road Satellite, **Ahmedabad** 380 015
  Phones: +91-079-26926233,   Rel: +91-079-32988717,   Fax: +91-079-26927094
  e-mail: jpamdvd@rediffmail.com

- 202 Batavia Chambers, 8 Kumara Krupa Road, Kumara Park East, **Bangalore** 560 001
  Phones: +91-80-22285971, +91-80-22382956,   Rel: +91-80-32714073
  Fax: +91-80-22281761   e-mail: jaypeemedpubbgl@eth.net

- 282 IIIrd Floor, Khaleel Shirazi Estate, Fountain Plaza, Pantheon Road, **Chennai** 600 008
  Phones: +91-44-28193265, +91-44-28194897,   Rel: +91-44-32972089
  Fax: +91-44-28193231   e-mail: jpchen@eth.net

- 4-2-1067/1-3, 1st Floor, Balaji Building, Ramkote Cross Road, **Hyderabad** 500 095
  Phones: +91-40-66610020, +91-40-24758498,   Rel:+91-40-32940929
  Fax:+91-40-24758499,   e-mail: jpmedpub@rediffmail.com

- No. 41/3098, B & B1, Kuruvi Building, St. Vincent Road, **Kochi** 682 018, Kerala
  Phones: +91-0484-4036109, +91-0484-2395739, +91-0484-2395740
  e-mail: jaypeekochi@rediffmail.com

- 1-A Indian Mirror Street, Wellington Square, **Kolkata** 700 013
  Phones: +91-33-22451926, +91-33-22276404, +91-33-22276415,   Rel: +91-33-32901926
  Fax: +91-33-22456075,   e-mail: jpbcal@dataone.in

- 106 Amit Industrial Estate, 61 Dr SS Rao Road, Near MGM Hospital, Parel, **Mumbai** 400 012
  Phones: +91-22-24124863, +91-22-24104532,   Rel: +91-22-32926896
  Fax: +91-22-24160828,   e-mail: jpmedpub@bom7.vsnl.net.in

- "KAMALPUSHPA" 38, Reshimbag, Opp. Mohota Science College
  Umred Road, **Nagpur** 440 009 (MS)
  Phones: Rel: 3245220,   Fax: 0712-2704275   e-mail: jaypeenagpur@dataone.in

Hysterectomy Made Easy

First Edition: **2007**
ISBN 81-8448-010-5

Typeset at JPBMP typesetting unit
Printed at Gopsons Papers Ltd., Noida.

PREFACE

Hysterectomy (abdominal or vaginal route) is usally done for various gynecological pathology. During this procedure there may be chance to cause hemorrhage or hematoma due to slipping or injugy to the uterine or ovarian artery. To tackle this hemorrhage there may be every chance to injure the ureter, bladder and rectum, etc. due to inexperience of handling the unwanted catastrophy.

To prevent this complication author had developed new approach ligation of uterine and ovarian artery prior to abdominal and vaginal hysterectomy procedures. This book is not only highlighted the anatomy of female pelvis and different operative techniques including its modification but also focussed the epidemiological survey, documentation and hormone replacement therapy, etc.

I hope contents of this book will definitely help gynecologists to tackle any complication arises during operative procedures.

I am very grateful to my son Indranil Dutta, medical student, wife Dr Banani Dutta and Sanjib Dutta for their help to prepare this book.

My sincere and heartiest thanks are due to M/s Jaypee Brothers Medical Publishers (P) Ltd., New Delhi, for publication of this book.

DK Dutta

Contents

CHAPTER 1

Abdominal Hysterectomy— A Historical Review

1768 : *Cavallini* performed hysterectomy on sheep and dogs.

1889 : *Stinson* was first to practice systematic ligation of ovarian and uterine vessels preliminary to hysterectomy operation.

1929 : *Richardson* originally described the technique of abdominal hysterectomy by applying clamp from above downwards.

1992 : *Dilip Kumar Dutta* performed ligation uterine artery prior to conventional hysterectomy procedure.

2000 : *Dilip Kumar Dutta* performed new techniques of abdominal hysterectomy-clampless.

2003 : *Dilip Kumar Dutta* demosntrated this technique at World Congress, Santiago (Chile).

2006 : *Dilip Kumar Dutta* demosntrated this technique at World Congress Kualalampur (Malaysia).

CHAPTER 2

The Anatomy of Female Pelvis

To any gynecological surgeon (pelvic surgeon) anatomical landmark of pelvis are important while performing a gynecologic operation which includes the planes and spaces in the pelvis, the close relationship between the urinary reproductive and gastrointestinal tracts,the vascular, lymphatic and collateral circulation of female pelvis and neuromuscular innervation and support of pelvic viscera.

THE PELVIC VISCERA

The female reproductive tract,occupies a unique position in pelvis, is developmentally interposed between bladder anteriorly and rectum posteriorly. Hence, to remove uterus from its location between the adjacent bladder and rectum requires not only surgical skill but an understanding of fascial planes, ligaments and vessels that involve the uterus and adjacent viscera (Fig. 2.1).

ANATOMY OF UTERUS

When the female pelvis is viewed from anterior and superior aspects the close approximation of sigmoid colon, the uterus and the bladder can be seen. The most anterior is the round ligament, which passes laterally and ventrally to reach the abdominal inguinal ring. The most posterior structure is the ovarian ligament which is attached to the posterior leaf of the broad ligament and extends from the uterine pole of the ovary to the side of the uterus just below the origin of the fallopian tube. Adjacent to the mesovarium is the suspensory ligaments of the ovary, the infundibulopelvic ligament, which extends laterally between the two layers of the broad ligament from the tubal extremity of the ovary to lateral pelvic wall. This

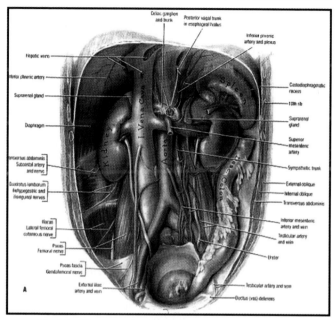

Fig. 2.1: Viscera and vessels of posterior abdominal wall

ligament forms the lateral portion of the free boundary of both broad ligaments. The central and most superior of these structures running in the upper border of the broad ligament is the fallopian (uterine) tube. The fallopian tube has four parts, the first of which is the infundibulum, a funnellike dilatation that opens into the abdominal cavity by way of the external ostium, which is surrounded by numerous diverging processes, the fimbriae.

ANATOMY OF THE BLADDER

The bladder is retroperitoneal viscus that is located behind the symphysis pubis and rests on the anterior portion of the urogenital diaphragm, vaginal fornix of the vagina. and lower uterine segment. The base of the bladder is closely related to the lower uterine segment and the anterior fornix of the vagina. The trigone of the bladder os contigious with the upper one-third of the vagina and anterior fornix, while the remainder of the bladder base rests intimately on the cervix and the inferior portion of the uterine segment.

The bladder has been opened for a views of lateral interior in the Figures 2.2 and 2.3. The three openings in the base of the bladder are the orifices of the two ureters and the urethra. The interuretic ridge is a slightly curved, transverse fold of the mucosa that extends between the two ureteral orifices and forms the superior boundary of the vesical trigone. The three angles of the trigone are represented by the orifices of urethra and the two ureters. This area is redder in color and is free from the folds that characterize the remainder of the bladder mucosa. The ureteral orifices are separated by 3 to 5 mm, depending on the contraction or distention of the bladder wall. The terminal ureters pass through vesical wall (5-7 mm) and into the bladder at the lateral and superior angles of the trigone. During their medial diversion into the trigone,the terminal 3 to 4 cm of the ureter passes along the anterior fornix from the position immediately adjacent to the lateral vaginal wall.

The trigone itself is approximately 2.5 to 3.0 cm in length from the internal uretral orifice to the interuveteric ridge. Since the length of the anterior vaginal wall is 8 cm or slightly more in adult female the superior margin of the trigone of the bladder is 1 cm or more in the adult female, the superior margin of the trigone of the bladder is 1 cm or more inferior to the apex of the vaginal fornix. Anatomically, it is important to understand that the

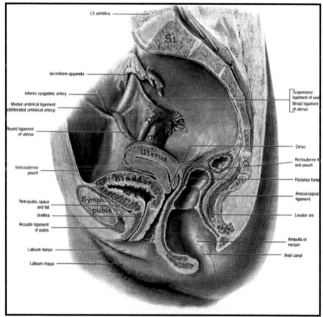

Fig. 2.2: Female pelvis: median section, lateral view

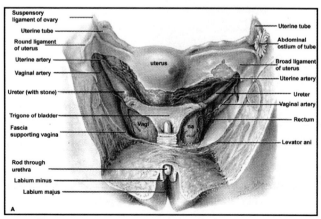

Fig. 2.3: Female pelvis: median sections anterior view

trigone rests on the upper one third of the vagina and anterior fornix.

ANATOMY OF THE URETER

The relationships of the abdominal and pelvic ureter are important. In general, the ureter measures approximately 25 to 30 cm in total length in the adult. The abdominal ureter is approximately 13 to 15 cm in length and courses retroperitoneally along the anteromedial aspect of the psoas muscle throughout its abdominal route to the pelvis (Fig. 2.4). The medial border of the right ureter lies in close approximation to the lateral margin of the vena cava. This has created some anatomical difficulty in dissecting the paracaval lymph nodes from the inferior vena cava and the necessitates the careful lateral retraction of the ureter, should a lymph node, dissection be performed in this region. The right ureter crosses the common illiacartery

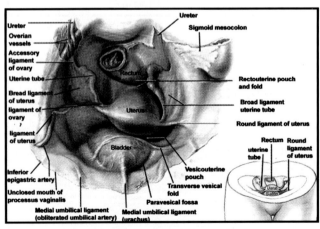

Fig. 2.4: Female true pelvis, superior view

at or just beyond its bifurcation. The pelvic ureter, which is approximately equal in length to the abdominal segment (13-15 cm) passes along the posterolateral aspect of the pelvis and anterior to the hypogastric artery. Here, it courses along the obturator muscle to the region in the greater sciatic notch to the level of the ischial spine. In this part of its course, the ureter lies in between the obturator nerve and the anterior division of the hypogastric artery on its lateral side and the peritoneum of the cul-de-sac of Douglas on its medial side. At this point, the ureter turns forward and medially, passing lateral to the uterosacral ligament, through the cardinal ligament and beneath the uterine artery and vein, approximately 1.5 to 2 cm lateral to the internal cervical os. It continues slightly medially for approximately 2 to 3 cm where it comes in close approximation to the anterior vaginal fornix and passes medially to enter the base of the bladder at the trigone. Its intramural (3 mm) and submucosal (7 mm) portions give a combined length to the bladder segment of the ureter of 1 cm or more. The ureter opens obliquely into the ureterovesical junction. The critical anatomical points where ureteral injury can occur include the juxtaposition of the ureter beneath the uterine artery, its medial course along the lower portion of the cardinal ligament and the anterior vaginal fornix before it enters the base of the bladder, its course along the base of the broad ligament just lateral to the uterosacral ligament, and its position along the medial aspect of the infundibulopelvic ligament where it crosses the pelvic brim (Figs 2.5 and 2.6).

ANATOMY OF SIGMOID COLON

The lower portion of the sigmoid colon passes medially into the midline of the pelvis, where it becomes closely

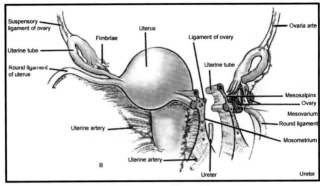

Fig. 2.5: Uterus and broad ligament

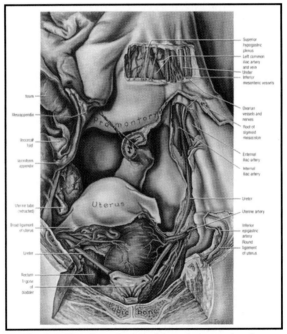

Fig. 2.6: Female ureter in pelvis, anterosuperior view

related to the uterus and vagina and is continuous with the rectum below the peritoneal reflection of the cul-de-sac of Douglas. The rectum is closely situated against the posterior fornix and the vaginal wall, from which it is separated by a thin layer of loose areolar tissue. The rectum passes through the posterior aspect of the pelvic floor, directly behind the urogenital diaphragm, where it is supported by the puborectalis portion of the levator ani muscles. It terminates in the anal canal and anus and serves principally as a reservoir for the fecal content of the lower colon prior to the voluntary fecal expulsion through the anal canal during the process of defecation. The anal canal is approximately 3 to 4 cm in length and serves as a flattened, empty conduit of the lower colon that terminates in the anus.This portion of the colon is bounded superiorly by the levator ani muscles and inferiorly by anus. Its principal function is in producing fecal continence.

Because of these favorable anatomical relationships, the rectum is injured infrequently during pelvic surgery in the ratio of approximately 1 to 4, as compared to the bladder (Fig. 2.7).

BLOOD SUPPLY TO THE PELVIS

It is very important and safe for gynecological surgeon to know the blood supply of different organs of the pelvis while performing the pelvic surgery.

Abdominal Aorta and Inferior Vena Cava

Abdominal aorta begins at the aortic hiatus of the diaphragm in front of the lower border of the last thoracic vertebrae. It descends along the front of the vertebral

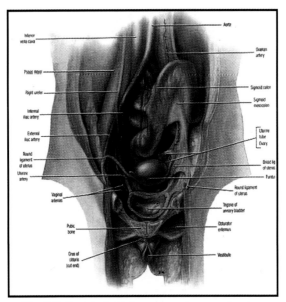

Fig. 2.7: Female genital organs, anterosuperior view

column, where it bifurcates at the fourth lumbar vertebrae and divides into the left and right common iliac arteries. The level on the abdominal wall of the aortic bifurcation at L4 is ator near umbilicus. An incision to permit the surgical approach to the lower portion of the aorta must be extended somewhat above the umbilicus. Infrequently, the aortic bifurcation may occur as high as the third lumbar vertebrae. Prior to its bifurcation, the abdominal aorta gives off two major branches that supply arterial blood to the pelvic viscera: the ovarian artery and the inferior mesenteric artery.

The right ovarian artery is seen to cross the anterior surface of the vena cava and the lower portion of the abdominal ureter, where it courses on the lateral side of the ureter to enter the pelvis through the infundibulo-pelvic ligament. In contrast, the left ovarian artery crosses the ureter immediately after arising from the anterolateral aspect of the abdominal aorta approximately 1 cm below the site of origin of renal artery and vein. The left ovarian artery courses along the lateral side of ureter to cross the bifurcation of the common iliac artery at the pelvic brim. It enters the infundibulopelvic ligament to supply the ovary and to communicate with an arcade that fuses with the uterine artery in the broad ligament. The course of the two ovarian veins is different. The left ovarian vein passes along the surface of the psoas muscle to drain into the left renal vein before the latter enters the vena cava. In contrast, the right ovarian vein passes along the infundibulopelvic ligament, crosses the pelvic brim, where it passes over the lower portion of the abdominal ureter with the ovarian artery, and ascends along the vena cava approximately 1 cm below the right renal vein. Enlargement and distention of the right ovarian vein during pregnancy has been associated with the dilatation of the abdominal ureter above the pelvic brim and have been questioned as factors causing right hydronephrosis during pregnancy.

The inferior mesenteric artery arises approximately 3 to 4 cm above the bifurcation of aorta and passes into the root of the mesentry of sigmoid colon, where it supplies the rectosigmoid colon through the superior hemorrhoidal artery, which communicates freely with the middle and inferior hemorrhoidal arteries.

At the aortic bifurcation, the right common iliac artery crosses over the proximal portion of the left common iliac vein before the left and right iliac veins give rise to the vena cava.

The right common iliac artery continues along the medial border of the psoas muscle to the pelvic brim, where it divides into the external iliac and hypogastric arteries. It continues obliquely and laterally along the medial border of the psoas muscle to pass below the medial portion of the inguinal ligament, where it continues as the femoral artery.

It is important to note that the right common iliac artery courses on the medial side of the common iliac vein near its proximal portion but deviates to the lateral side of external iliac vein as it approaches the femoral canal. These anatomical relationships are important during the dissection of the lymphatics of the external and common iliac vessels because the thin walls of the iliac veins may be traumatised easily if their precise boundaries are not fully appreciated. The left common and external iliac artery, however remain on the lateral side of the corresponding iliac vein at all times throughout their course along the pelvic brim before the external iliac artery and vein enter the femoral canal. Therefore, the lateral aspect of the left common and external iliac artery can be dissected without danger of trauma to the vein, which always courses along the medial side of artery. The right common iliac artery is usually slightly longer than the left and courses more obliquely across the body of last lumbar vertebrae. Immediately lateral to its origin is the right common iliac vein. The left common iliac artery continues along the medial border of the psoas muscle on the lateral side of left common iliac vein before dividing into the external iliac and hypogastric arteries near the lumbosacral joint. The external iliac artery provides no arterial blood directly to the pelvis except for the infrequent anomalous obturator artery that may arise from its distal end. When this anomaly occurs, there is a important source of collateral circulation with the hypogastric artery.

The middle sacral artery arises from the posteroinferior aspect of the aorta at its bifurcation and courses under the left common iliac vein to pass over L5 before emerging over the pelvic brim and along the anterior surface of the sacrum together with the presacral nerve. The middle sacral vein(s) courses over the sacral vertebrae and enters the inferior vena cava at its origin from the common iliac veins.

The hypogastric artery provides the blood supply to the pelvic viscera and musculature. It continues through the ischiorectal fossa as the internal pudendal artery to the perineum and vulva, where it extends within the labia to reach the urogenital diaphragm and the clitoris. For descriptive purpose, the hypogastric artery may be divided into an anterior and posterior trunk. The posterior division gives off parietal branches only, while the anterior branches gives off mainly visceral branches but also some parietal branches.

Internal Pudendal

The anterior division gives off its most medial visceral branch, the uterine artery, prior to continuing along the medial aspect of the paravesical space to supply the superior and inferior vesical branches to the bladder. The bladder obtains its superior vesical branch from the segment of the anterior division that continues as the obliterated umbilical artery and passes along the inferior surface of the rectus muscle to insert in the umbilicus along with the urachus from the bladder. The branches of the anterior division supply the uterus, the uterine tube, the vagina, the bladder. The uterine artery passes through the base of the broad ligament, where it deviates sharply medially along with the uterine vein to course over the ureter and to send collateral branches to the fundus, where it forms a collateral branches to the fundus, where it forms a collateral anchor with the ovarian artery. The uterine artery also gives off decending branches to the cervix and vagina.

The inferior vesical artery usually arises from the anterior division of the hypogastric artery, either separately or as a branch from the cervical or vaginal artery. It anastomoses freely with the middle and superior vesical arteries. In addition to the visceral branches, the anterior division gives origin to three parietal branches: the obturator, the internal pudendal, and the inferior gluteal arteries. The obturator artery is the most proximal parietal branch of the anterior division and runs forward and posteriorly into the base of the obturator space, where it courses along with obturator nerve above it and the obturator vein below, to leave the pelvis through the obturator foramen. The terminal portion of the anterior division of the hypogastric artery continues as the internal pudendal artery.

The bladder is supplied by the superior, the middle, and the inferior vesical arteries. The superior vesical artery arises from the umbilical artery,which is obliterated distal to point of branching, it supplies the superior surface of the bladder and anastomoses with the other vesical arteries. The middle vesical artery may arise from either the umbilical artery or from one of the branches of the superior vesical. The inferior vesical usually arises from the anterior trunk of the hypogastric or as a branch from the cervical or vaginal artery and is distributed to the base of the bladder.

The rectosigmoid colon is supplied by three arteries: the superior haemorrhoidal which continues from the inferior mesenteric artery: the middle haemorrhoidal from the anterior trunk of the hypogastric: and the inferior hemorrhoidal, which arises from the internal pudendal artery. These haemorrhoidal vessels anastomose freely. Any compromise of the the blood supply to the rectum from any one of these vessels is easily compensated for by a rich collateral circulation from other vessels.

All the branches of the posterior division of the hypogastric artery are parietal. They include the illiolumbar, the lateral sacral, and the superior gluteal arteries. The illiolumbar artery originates most proximately from the posterior division of the hypogastric artery and immediately divides into lumbar and iliac branches. The lateral sacral artery may be paired or may arise as a single trunk, giving branches to the first, second, third, and fourth anterior sacral foramina. Some of the branches of the lateral sacral artery communicate directly with branches from middle sacral artery. The superior gluteal artery, which is the third and largest branch of the posterior division of hypogastric, passes posteriorly, usually between the first sacral nerve and the lumbosacral trunk and continues posteriorly, where it leaves the pelvis through the greater sciatic foramen above the piriformis muscle.

COLLATERAL ARTERIAL CIRCULATION OF THE FEMALE PELVIS

The collateral circulation of the female pelvis is extensive and provides a variety of intercommunicating sources of arterial blood from various sites along the arterial tree. These collateral vessels anastomose with the hypogastric artery and the blood supply to the uterus through a number of circuitous arterial pathways in the pelvis. During a difficult hysterectomy, the collateral circulation may create problem in receiving adequate haemostasis. Therefore, it is important to have a clear understanding of the various extrapelvic arteries that communicate with the pelvic circulation (Fig. 2.8).

The collateral circulation of the pelvis may be divided into three main arterial groups: those vessels that communicate with the branches from the aorta; those that communicate with the branches from the external iliac

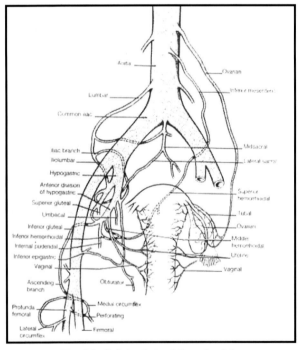

Fig. 2.8: Collateral circulation of pelvis

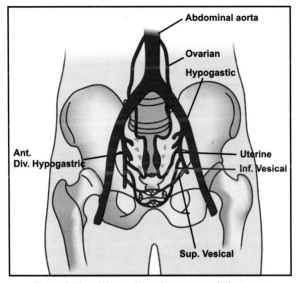

Fig. 2.9: Arterial arcade and anastomosis between
ovarian and uterine arteries

artery; and those that communicate with the branches
from the femoral artery (Figs 2.9 to 2.15).

NERVE SUPPLY TO THE PELVIS

The pelvic organs are innervated by both sympathetic and
parasympathetic nerves. The abdominal sympathetic
nerves pass to the pelvis through four pathways:(1) some
fibers follow the abdominal sympathetic chain into the
pelvis (2) other fibers traverse the sympathetic plexus with
the ovarian and (3) superior hemorrhoidal vessels; while
(4) most of the sympathetic fibers enter the para-aortic
plexus and leave the abdomen as the hypogastric

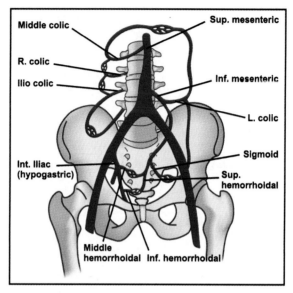

Fig. 2.10: Collateral circulation of inferior mesenteric artery to branches of hypogastric artery from superior hemorrhoidal to middle and inferior hemorrhoidal arteries

(presacral) plexus, principally from spinal cord levels LI through L4.

The presacral plexus divides into right and left parts to enter the two pelvic nerve bundles. These presacral nerves pass deep into the pelvis to become the part of the pelvic plexus. The deep pelvic plexus is further divided into anterior subdivision, which provides a vesical plexus where it innervates the base of the bladder and the urethra, and a posterior division, which sends fibers to the uterine fundus, cervix, vagina, rectosigmoid colon, and the anal canal. The parasympathetic nerves enter the pelvis

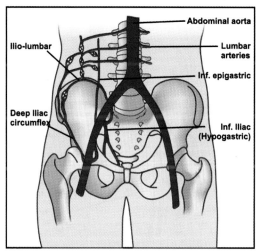

Fig. 2.11: Collateral circulation of aorta and hypogastric arteries through lumbar and iliolumbar anastomoses

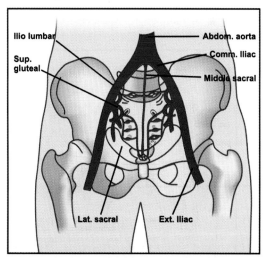

Fig. 2.12: Anastomosis of middle sacral artery from aorta with hypogastric branches, including lateral sacral and iliolumbar arteries

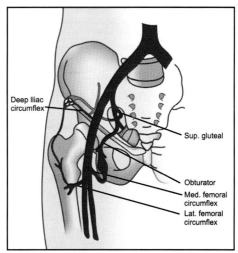

Fig. 2.13: Collateral arterial circulation between external iliac and hypogastric arteries through anastomoses with iliolumbar and superior gluteal arteries. Note anastomoses from medial and lateral femoral circumflex vessels with obturator and superior gluteal branches of hypogastric artery

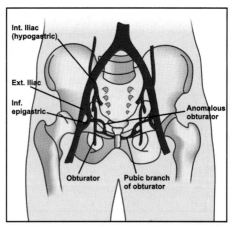

Fig. 2.14: Anastomosis of external iliac and hypogastric arteries through obturator originating anomalously from inferior epigastric artery

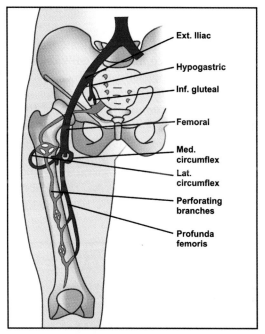

Fig. 2.15: Anastomoses of deep medial and lateral femoral circumflex arteries around hip joint to posterior division inferior gluteal of hypogastric artery

through the second, third and fourth sacral nerves (S2,S3,S4) and their preganglionic fibres are distributed to the pelvic organs through the pelvic nerve plexus. This plexus also receives sympathetic postganglionic fibres that originate in the spinal cord levels L1 through L4 and reach the pelvis by described pathways. These sympathetic fibers pass through the hypogastric plexus, and both the sympathetic and parasympathetic nerves enter the uterus from within the broad ligaments, as well as along the utersacral ligaments.

The major sensory nerves from the pelvic viscera are carried along the sympathetic nerve plexus to reach their origin in the spinal cord, principally along L2 to L4. For this reason, uterine discomfort is usually registered in the lower abdomen or hypogastrium, which is regional area innervated by the lumbar nerves. This neurologic phenomenon is understandable in view of the fact that the uterus arose, embryologically, from the mesothelium of the abdominal cavity, along the developing lumbar vertebrae. Pain stimuli originating from the cervix are usually registered through the sacral sympathetic chain and conducted through the uterosacral ligaments to the sacral sympathetic plexus from S2, S3, and S4. Therefore,

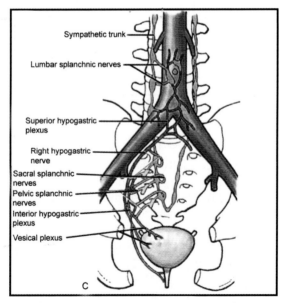

Fig. 2.16: Sympathetic nerve supply to the pelvis

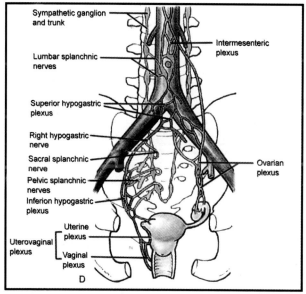

Fig. 2.17: Parasympathetic nerve supply to the pelvis

pain from the cervix is frequently referred to the lumbo-sacral region (Figs 2.16 to 2.18).

BIBLIOGRAPHY

1. Bossy J. Atlas of Neuroanatomy and Special Sense Organs Philedelphia, WB Saunders,1970.
2. Burchell RC. Physiology of Internal Illiac Artery Ligation, J Obstet Gynaecol Br Commw 1968;75:642.
3. Curtis AH,Anson BJ, Ashley FL, et al. The Anatomy of Pelvic Autonomic Nerves In Relation to Gynaecology 1942;75:743.
4. Figge FHJ(Ed): Sabotta's Atlas of Human Anatomy, 8th Edition,Vol 1-3 New York, Hafner,1962.
5. Georgy FM: Femoral neuropathy following abdominal, hysterectomy. Am J Obstet Gynaecol, 1975:123:819.

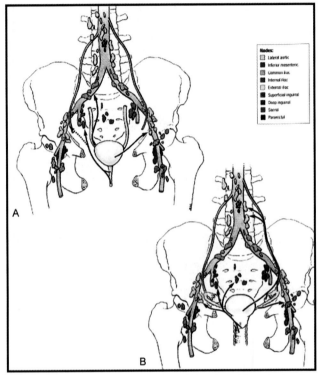

Figs 2.18A and B: Lymphatic drainage of female pelvis, anterior views. A. Uterus, urinary bladder, and urethra. B. Uterus, vagina, uterine tubes, and ovaries

6. Goss CM (Ed): Gray's Anatomy of Human Body, 29th Edition Philadelphia, Lea And Febiger,1973.
7. Hopper CL,Baker JB: Bilateral Femoral Neuropathy Complicating Vaginal Hysterectomy, Obstet Gynaecol 1968:32:543.
8. Krantz KE: Anatomy of Female Reproductive System.in Benson RC(Ed): Current Obstetrics and Gynaecologic Diagnosis and Treatment, 2nd Ed Los Altos,Calif, Lange Medical Publications, 1978
9. Kuhn RJP, Hollyock VE: Observations on the Anatomy of the Rectovaginal Pouch and Septum. Obstet Gynaecol 1982:59;445.

CHAPTER 3

Informed Consent for Hysterectomy Operation

Six universal agreement for informed consent
- Diagnosis
- Nature and purpose of the procedure
- Risks of the procedure
- Likely hood of success
- Resonable alternatives
- Prognosis if the treatment is refused

GUIDELINES REGARDING INFORMED CONSENT

1. The obligation to obtain the informed consent of a woman before any medical intervention is undertaken derives from respect for her fundamental human rights. These rights have been widely agreed on and are laid down in such documents as the Universal Declaration of Human Rights (1948), the twin International Coverants on Civil and Political Rights and Economics, Social and Cultural Rights (1975), the International Convention on the Elimination of all forms of Discrimination Against Women (1979), Sexual and Reproductive Human Rights have also been identified by the International Conference on Population in Cairo (1994), and re-affirmed by the Fourth World Conference on Women in Beijing(1995).

2. The flooring definition (1) of informed consent flows from these human rights and endorsed by the FIGO Committee for the Study of Ethical Aspects of Human Reproduction.

   "Informed consent is a consent obtained freely, without threats or improper inducements, after appropriate disclosure to the patient of adequate and understandable information in a form and language understood by the patient on:

   a. the diagnostic assessment

    b. the purpose, method, likely duration and expected benefit of the proposed treatment

    c. alternative modes of treatment, including those less intrusive, and

    d. possible pain or discomfort, risks and side-effects of the proposed treatment.

3. Although these criteria are clear, to implement them may be difficult and time consuming, for example where women have little education, of where very unequal power relationships in a societs initiate against women's selt determination. Nevertheless these difficulties not absolve physician s caring for women from pursuing fulfilment of these criteria for informed consent. Only the woman can decide if the benefits to her of a procedure are worth the risks and discomfort she may undergo. Even if, for exampple other family members feel they should make the decision, it is the ethical obligation of the physician to ensure her human right of self determination is met by the process of communication theat procedures any informed consent.

4. It is important to keep in mind the fact that informed consent is not a signature but a process of communication and interaction.

5. The opinion of children or adolescents on a medical intervention should be assessed within the limitation posed by their level of development, age or understanding.

6. Even if a woman is unable to decide for herself because of mental incapacity or mental retardation, nevertheless she must be involved in the decision-making process to the fullest extent her capacity allows and her best interests must be taken into account.

7. If physicians for reason of their own religious or other beliefs do not wish to fulfil the above criteria for

informed consent because they do no want to give information on some alternatives; they have, as a matter of respect for their patient's human rights, an ethical obligation to make an appropriate referral so she may obtain the full information necessary to make a valid choice.

*Note 1: UN Resoultion on Principles for the Protection of Persons with Mental Illness and for the Improvement of Mental Health Care 11.2, **Jerusalem, 1995***

INFORMED CONSENT AND REQUEST FOR HYSTERECTOMY

I, ..., request Dr. ....and his/her associates/assistants to perform upon me: (Circle procedure of choice)
1. Removal of uterus (womb)
2. Possible removal of tubes and/or ovaries
3. Possible removal of appendix

Diagnosis and Procedure; The following has been explained to me in general terms and I understand that:

May condition has been diagnosed as:_____
The nature of the procedure is: _____
The purpose of this procedure is to: _____

General risk of surgery: As a result of the performance of this procedure there may be general risks involved such as: *Infection, Allergic Reaction, Disfiguring Scar, Severe Loss of Blood, Function of any Limb of Organ, Paralysis, Paraplegia or Quadriplegia, Brain Damage, Cardiac Arrest or Death.* In addition to these general risks, there may be other possible risks involved in this procedure. These risks and/or complications may include but are not limited to such complications as:

1. Injury to bowel, biadder, or ureter, which could result in a fistula formaiton, an opening between bowel, bladder, ureter, vagina and/or skin.
2. Need for a colostomy or a second operation to repair any of the above injuries.
3. Possible need for hormones.
4. Blood loss necessitating transfusion, which carries the risk of exposure to AIDS of the hepatitis virus.
5. Pelvic pain due to adhesions, scar tissue, or residual ovary.

Likelihood of Success: The likelihood of success of the above procedure is () Good, () Fair, () Poor

Prognosis: If I choose not to have the hysterectomy, my prognosis (future medical condition) is:

_____

Alternative forms of treatment such as:
1. Do nothing and accept the consequences of my present condition.
2. Dilatation and curettage procedure, laser treatment, or removal of fibroid tumors.
3. Hormone therapy.

These alternative treatments have been explained tome and I have elected this surgical procedure as my method of treatment.

I understand and accept that during the procedure unexpected or unforeseen circumstances may make it necessary to do an extension of the original procedure of another procedure that is not named above. I request that Dr .... and associates or assistants of his/her choice perform those procedure that they judge to be necessary.

By signing this form. I acknowledge that I have read or had this form read and explained to me and that I fully understand its contents.

I have been given ample opportunity to ask questions and any questions I have asked have been answered ro explained in a statisfactory manner. All blands or statements requiring completion manner. All blanks or statements requiring completion were filled in and all statements with which I disagree were marked out before i signed this form.

I accept that medicine is not an exact science and understand that no guarantees can be given as to the results. Understanding these limitations, I request that Dr ...... and his/her associates/assistants to proceed with surgery.

_____

Witness

_____

Person giving consent

_____

Relationship to patient if not the patient

_____

Patient unable to sign because of:

Date _____

Additoinal materials used, if any, during the informed consent process for this procedure include:

Date: _____   Witness: _____

CHAPTER 4

Preoperative Evaluation

1. *History*—Age, parity, socioeconomic status, medical, surgical, family, immunization, obstetrical, gynecological, drug, allergy.

2. *General health examination*—Pulse, pallor, edema, BP, obesity, CVS, RS, CNS, thyroid.

3. *Breast examination*—To see symmetry, size, condition of nipples, the presence of gross laisons and the presence of discharge. Any suspicious laisons is subjected for further evaluation by mammography, USG, aspiration, and/or biopsy to confirm the existence of a significant breast pathology.

4. *Abdominal examination*—Visual inspection, palpation, percussion and auscultation are useful method to find and differentiate various altered pathology. When any finding are conflicting or in conclusive, imaging procedure – like USG, CT Scan or MRI are helpful in completing the assessment of an abnormal abdominal examination.

5. *Pervaginal examination*—By (a) Speculum examination- vaginal, cervical pathology can be detected. In any suspicion (i) Pap smear from cervix or vagina or (ii) lugol's iodine on (ii) colposcopy examination to be instituted. (b) Bimanual examination – is to be done by the abdominal vaginal route for position, size, motility irregularity, Tenderness in motion. It also help to find out any adenexal pathology.

6. *Per recial examination*—In combination with vaginal examination are usually useful for evaluating the broad and between sacral ligaments, cul-de-sac of Douglus, uterus and adenexa. When pelvic findings are doubtful or inclusive imaging techniques are may be helpful in determining the preoperative diagnosis.

7. *Examination under anesthesia (EUA)*—When pervaginal, per-rectal examination and imaging techniques

or unavailable – EUA can be performed before final decision for or against gynecological surgery is made.

8. *Laboratory test*—Include (a) Blood Count with hemoglobin , hemotocrit (b) coagulation status (c) group and Rh factor (d) Kidney function test – urea, creatinine , uric acid (e) Liver function test (f) Blood Sugar, GTT (g) Urinalysis (h) Chest X-ray (i) Electrocardiogram.

9. *Assessment by anesthesiologist*—To find out the risk of category of patient and types of surgical procedure and length of time of operation.

10. *Preoperative*—Antibiotic, control of serum blood glucose levels in all diabetic patient, control of RTI and others.

11. *Antiseptic*—Dressing to whole abdomen including lumbosacral region preoperative day.

12. *Operative day*—Cleaning of abdomen and vagina, catheterization of bladder, maintenance of IV fluid.

13. Preoperative, vaginal application of estrogen cream in old women undergoing VH.

CHAPTER 5

Postoperative Evaluation

Basic idea a) to prevent (1) Thromboembolism, (2) Bleeding from vault (3) Infection (4) Hypoventilation (5) Acute ventilator failure (6) Acute respiratory distress syndrome (7) Pneumonia (8) Oliguria or anuria. b)To maintain nutrition and early ambulation.

Postoperative Orders

- Intravenous fluid
- Indwelling catheter on in selected cases.
- Antibiotic.
- Anti emetic.
- Pain medication.
- Input and output chart.
- Oxygenation.
- Monitoring of pulse, BP, respirator, temperature.
- Encourage deep breathing.
- Early ambulatory.
- Venous thrombosis prophylaxis.
- Amino acid drip in poor moribund patient.
- Tubal feeding in selected cases.
- Nasogastric tube in selected case.
- Vaginal irrigation by antiseptic.
- Avoid constipation, cough.
- Use commode system.
- Maintain hygiene.

CHAPTER 6

Abdominal Incision: Advantages and Disadvantages

Various types of incisions for abdominal hysterectomy and their comparative advantages and disadvantages are shown in Figure 6.1.

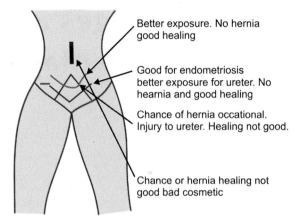

Better exposure. No hernia good healing

Good for endometriosis better exposure for ureter. No hearnia and good healing

Chance of hernia occasional. Injury to ureter. Healing not good.

Chance or hernia healing not good bad cosmetic

Fig. 6.1: Various types of incision for abdominal hysterectomy operation

CHAPTER 7

Controvercies of Different Procedures of Hysterectomy

TOTAL VERSUS SUBTOTAL ABDOMINAL HYSTERECTOMY

Abdominal hysterectomy, both total and subtotal, had become a relatively safe operation in the hands of a competent gynecologist. In the past two decades, total hysterectomy has been accepted as the preferred method of removal of the uterus.

To compare the two procedures, one should balance the advantages of removal of the cervix against the possibilities of an increased morbidity and mortality for the total operation. To some extent, this is difficult to do because subtotal abdominal hysterectomy is now performed only in patients with very serious pelvic disease. Therefore, as one might expect, postoperative mortality and morbidity from total abdominal hysterectomy, but for reasons that have nothing to do with differences in the operative technique. The incidence of the development of carcinoma is no greater in the retained stump than in the cervix of the intact uterus. Since the incidence of cervical carcinoma in a cervix that has had repeated cytologic evaluation is extremely low, the major disadvantages of the retained cervix is the requirement for continued cytologic follow-up. While there is a recognized false negative rate of vaginal cytology of approximately 10 to 15%, repeated cytologic study and clinical evaluation of the figure. Therefore, the rationale for the removal of the cervix must be based on the disease process that necessitates the hysterectomy and on the risk of complications that my result from attempting to remove the cervix from its anatomical location between the bladder above, the rectum below, and the ureters on each side.

The indications for subtotal hysterectomy should be based solely on the surgical risk of this added procedure, since the current indications for removal of the uterus are for a total hysterectomy. Subtotal hysterectomy is performed in such cases as severe pelvic inflammatory disease, advanced endometriosis, ovarian cancer, and other conditions in which pelvic anatomy can not be clearly defined. The number of patients with carcinoma developing in a cervical stump has been reduced significantly in recent years, it is unfortunate that there are still women who die of this disease when it could have been avoided by spending a few extra minutes to do a total rather than subtotal hysterectomy. Although there is a minimal increase in the risk of vesicovaginal or rectovaginal fistula and ureteral injury with removal of the cervix, none of these complications should occur, especially in the absence of significant pelvic disease, if proper surgical technique is used. When the danger of removing the cervix exceeds the danger of leaving it in should the subtotal operation be done.

OVARIAN MANAGEMENT AT HYSTERECTOMY

In the early twentieth century, as ovarian physiology began to be understood, an era of ovarian conservation began. At the same time, however, the concept of prophylactic surgery (as in prophylactic removal of the appendix and cervix) was gaining acceptance. Gynecologic surgeons, frustrated mostly by the difficulty of diagnosing and curing ovarian cancer, debated the merits of prophylactic removal of normal ovaries in premenopausal and postmenopausal women at the time of hysterectomy.

There are still no uniformly acceptable and established criteria for removal or retention of normal. When normal ovaries are conserved at the time of abdominal hysterectomy in premenopausal women, normal hormonal function will continue unaltered in cyclic fashion in almost all until the natural age of the menopause, at which time they time, they will cease to produce 17-b estradiol and progesterone. Most of the surgeon felt that normal ovarian function continues after hysterectomy with no evidence of altered arrangement of the follicular or corpus luteum development, maturation, or regression and no evidence of detectable changes in the ovarian stroma conducted that ovaries conserved after hysterectomy may continue to function for more than 15 years after hysterectomy. Since the ovary may not be the only source of estrogen affecting vaginal cytology, it has been necessary to confirm these findings with endocrine assays. Ovarian function was monitored by weekly urinary estrogen and pregnanediol determinations for periods of 4 to 6 weeks at intervals for up to 2.5 years.

If the ovary is to be conserved when hysterectomy is done, every attempt should be made to preserve its blood supply. The infundibulopelvic ligament containing the ovarian vessels must not be twisted or stretched. Clamps that are used to separate the ovary from the uterus should be placed as close to the uterine corpus as possible so that the arcade of vessels in the mesosalpinx that supply the ovary will not be interfered with. Normal tubes should be left with the ovary. Attempts to remove the tube could interfere with ovarian blood supply. Regarding the general option is that the uterine artery supplies the medical half of the ovary and the medial two-thirds of the fallopian tube, the rest of the blood supply coming from the ovarian artery. The distribution of these arteries, however, shows great variation, ranging from cases in which the ovarian artery supplies the entire tube and ovary to cases in which the blood supply of these organs is solely derived from the uterine artery. If a significant portion of the blood supply to the ovary is derived from the uterine artery, continued normal ovarian function might not be possible after a hysterectomy because of inadequate blood supply.

A permanent disturbance of blood flow to the ovary at the time of hysterectomy may explain the occurrence of the so-called residual ovary syndrome. Data suggest that 1 to 2% of patients who have one or both ovaries conserved at the time of hysterectomy will subsequently require operation for a problem with an ovary or tube.

The major risk of ovarian conservation at the time of hysterectomy is the risk that ovarian cancer, an admittedly devastating disease, will develop subsequently. Ovarian cancer remains one of the most lethal tumors of the female reproductive tract. There is no evidence to suggest that retained ovaries have a greater risk of neoplasia than do ovaries attached to an intact uterus, the gynecologist must accept the responsibility of assuring the patient that the continued hormonal function of the ovary has greater importance to the patient than the small risk of subsequent ovarian neoplasm.

The conclusion is that, since the incidence of ovarian cancer after hysterectomy is 0.1% of all females, even universally practiced prophylactic oophorectomy would not reduce the incidence significantly. Those who advocates of oophorectomy, expressed the belief that prophylactic oophorectomy cannot be justified on the basis of its effect in reducing the incidence of ovarian malignancy. Some surgeons are of the opinion that the problem of ovarian cancer subsequent to hysterectomy can be solved by conservation of only one ovary instead of two, apparently feeling that the incidence of subsequent ovarian cancer will be reduced by 50%. There is no statistical data to support this view. Realistically, to retain one ovary is to retain 100% of the malignant potential of both ovaries. It has been shown that the incidence of anovulatory cycle increases and that menopause occurs at an earlier age if only one ovary is conserved. When it comes to the question of conservation of normal ovarian function, two normal ovaries are better than one. By conserving two normal ovaries, the incidence of subsequent ovarian cancer is not known to be increased.

After hysterectomy, the role of the ovaries in the process of reproduction is irrelevant. However, the ovaries of premenopausal women play an active role in many basic metabolic processes throughout the body through secretion of estrogen, progesterone, and androgens. Ovarian hormones influence protein, calcium, bone, potassium and carbohydrate metabolism, among others. The absence of ovarian function over a period of years has been implicated in the pathogenesis of osteoporosis, coronary artery disease, and cerebrovascular accidents. There is evidence from bone densitometry and other studies that patients with premature castration of more than ten years before expected menopause have a higher incidence of osteoporosis and coronary artery disease. Yet, there are many other interrelated factors that influence the development of these diseases.

The question of ovarian hormonal replacement for the surgically castrated premenopausal women is a complicated one. Such replacement is not always well tolerated and certainly cannot and should not be depended upon to replace the useful function of normal ovaries to such an extent that premenopausal patients can be routinely castrated when abdominal hysterectomy is done.

The decision to remove the normal ovaries of a premenopausal woman is undergoing hysterectomy or to conserve their function, presents a difficult choice for the thoughtful gynecologic surgeon. It is difficult to believe that a remenopausal woman in any way, either physically or psychologically, by removing her normal ovaries. Evidence suggests that the grossly normal ovaries of premenopausal women should be conserved when hysterectomy is done. Although a decision to leave in or remove the ovaries should be based on an assessment of their functional status rather than on some arbitrary age, prophylactic oophorectomy is advised at the time of abdominal hysterectomy is advised at the time of abdominal hysterectomy in women who are within 1 or 2 years of the mean age of menopause (age 51). Normal ovaries should always be removed when abdominal hysterectomy is done on the postmenopausal woman.

Families with history of malignancy one often encounters women with early-onset ovarian carcinoma as well as one or more of the cardinal tumors of the family cancer syndrome, namely, endometrial, breast, and colonic carcinoma that primary carcinoma of the ovary is five times more frequent among women with previous carcinoma of the colon and rectum. A similar increase in the frequency of ovarian malignancy has been found in patients with breast carcinoma. Ovarian neoplasia is more common in the presence of the Peutz-Jeghers syndrome. Therefore, bilateral prophylactic oophorectomy should be done when hysterectomy is indicated in premenopausal patients with the Peutz-Jeghers syndrome; with a personal history of breast, colon, or rectal cancer; or with a strong family history of ovarian cancer. Unfortunately, prophylactic oophorectomy in women who have a high genetic risk for ovarian malignancy will not always accomplish the protection desired. In cancer-prone families, the susceptible tissue is not limited to the ovary but also includes other derivatives of the celomic epthelium, from which primary peritoneal neoplasms may arise following prophylactic oophorectomy. Ovarian cancer with intra-abdominal spread may actually represent multicentric neoplasia derived from the embryonic mesothelium or celomic epithelium. The peritoneum and the germinal epithelium. The peritoneum and the germinal epithelium of the ovary have a common embryologic origin.

With few exceptions, both ovaries should be removed in postmenopausal and premenopausal patients with endometrial and ovarian malignancy. Young women who have radical abdominal hysterectomy and bilateral lymphadenectomy for early invasive cervical cancer may have both normal ovaries conserved. When an ovary is severely involved by a tumor, cyst, infection, adhesions, or endometriosis, or when its blood supply is compromised, it should be removed. If an ovarian cystectomy is done, the ovary should be meticulously repaired with fine suture material to eliminate interstitial dead space and minimize adhesions. If more than two-thirds of the ovarian parenchyma has been removed, the entire ovary should be removed. During vaginal hysterectomy, the ovaries are examined but generally are not removed vaginally in the premenopausal patient. If the ovaries are accessible, the same guidelines for prophylactic oophorectomy should apply to the menopausal and postmenopausal patient at the time of vaginal hysterectomy. If it is important to remove the ovaries because of gross pathology or to resect an ovarian lesion, it should usually be done through an abdominal incision.

If a bilateral oophorectomy is done, whether for prophylactic reasons or because of pathology of the ovaries or uterus, the ovaries should be removed completely.

ABDOMINAL HYSTERECTOMY VERSUS VAGINAL HYSTERECTOMY

Abdominal hysterectomy that are emerging recently regarding the route of choice of operation to perform hysterectomy either by abdominal or by vaginal route. Vaginal route is found to be better choice than that of abdominal route as because (i) minimally invasive surgical technique (ii) less operative time (iii) reduction of hospital stay (iv) minimal blood loss (v) minimal operative and postoperative complications (vi) reduction of maternal mortality and morbidity. Although in case of severe endometriosis, pelvic adhesion, big ovarian tumor (VH is contraindicated) here choice of route is abdominal.

Vaginal hysterectomy vs Laparoscopic assisted vaginal hysterectomy (LAVH). Vaginal hysterectomy is the better route of choice (both non-descend and on descend uterus) than that of LAVH as because in LAVH there is increasing incidence of pelvic structural damage to(a) ureter (b) nerve plexus (c) bladder (d) vessels (e) postoperative morbidity.

CHAPTER 8

Cesarean Hysterectomy

Cesarean hysterectomy or postpartum hysterectomy is often an emergency procedure. Hemorrhage arising postpartum due to placenta acreta/increta/percreta, uterine atony or uterine rupture/perforation often compels a surgeon to do hysterectomy at the same sitting. Rarely in our modern practice cesarean hysterectomy may be indicated in severe infection or huge fibroid obstructing lower segment closure. Horatio R Storer in Boston performed the first cesarean hysterectomy in 1868.[1] The patient had a large lower segment fibroid, the baby was stillborn and the mother died 3 days later. Porro introduced the subtotal or supracervical hysterectomy in 1876 and at that time it made a remarkable difference to the mortality rate associated with such surgeries.[2] The incidence of such procedure varies in different parts of the world. In modern obstetrics with introduction of safer techniques of uterine artery ligation and more recently uterine artery embolisation the need for performing hysterectomy for uncontrolled bleeding needs to be reviewed. Still it remains as life saving procedure and obstetricians should be familiar with it. Review of obstetric hysterectomy at Ramathibodi Hospital, Bangkok[3] showed an incidence of 1 in 875 deliveries (91% emergency) while the incidence at Sapporo Medical University School of Medicine, Japan was 1 in 6,978 deliveries (0.014%).[4]

INDICATIONS

1. Uncontrolled hemorrhage
2. Rupture uterus
3. Abnormal placentation
4. Fibroids in uterus
5. Severe infections
6. Certain cases of carcinoma cervix
7. Failure of internal iliac-artery ligation to control hemorrhage.

RISK FACTORS

Cesarean delivery, prior cesarean delivery, placenta accreta and uterine atony have been identified as risk factors for emergency peri-partum hysterectomy and abnormal placentation is the primary cause of cesarean hysterectomy.

The combination of prior cesarean section and placenta previa is an especially ominous risk factor for emergency postpartum hysterectomy and life-threatening bleeding following placental removal.

PROCEDURE

The greatest problem is in *deciding* to do hysterectomy and not so much in performing the surgery. Various guidelines suggest that one should resort to hysterectomy *sooner rather than later* (especially in cases of placenta accreta or uterine rupture). If anticipated from before a midline incision is most suitable. But in case the need arises as an emergency the pfannenstiel's incision can be increased as a "smile". The rectus muscles if required can be reflected from their pubic insertion. Rarely one may need to make a T incision but this must be discouraged as such incisions heal poorly. As this surgery is done in emergency, simple, rapid and safe surgical techniques should be used. Ligation of uterine arteries (Dutta's technique) in both side is done as a first step to be followed by tying of mesosalpinx, fallopian tube utero ovarian ligament, round ligament (B) either by vicryl I-o or catgut suture. Subsequently because of congestion and friablity the round ligaments are again bilaterally clamped with double Heaney hysterectomy clamps, divided and suture ligated. The medial clamps help in preventing back bleeding and also can be used by assistant to apply upward traction of the uterus. The next step is to clamp utero-ovarian ligament and fallopian tubes, which are divided and sutured. Since bleeding is a major problem in these cases clamping of all major vascular pedicles is found to be better. A window is created in the broad ligament and adenexa are divided from the uterus. No 1 chromic catgut is most suitable as thinner catgut can cut through edematous tissue. The broad ligament is skeletonised by sharp dissection and progressively dissected from the uterus by serially placing clamps and suture ligating all pedicles till uterine artery is reached which is also divided and ligated. The lower segment in such cases is usually flaccid and dilated and it is difficult to externally palpate and determine lower edge of the cervix. Therefore sometimes a supposedly subtotal operation turns out to be total and *vice versa.* Once the uterine arteries are controlled the uterus is simple best-excised supracervically and this improves the exposure of the remaining cervix. If at this stage the patient is not hemodynamically stable the procedure can be terminated here. To remove cervix completely the tissues are then held with allies forceps, applied traction and dissected out. Kocher clamps are applied on the lateral edges and cardinal and uterosacral ligaments are progressively isolated and suture ligated till the edge of the cervix is reached. The cervix is then removed by circumferentially cutting the vagina. Meticulous attention to hemostais is required as most recurrent bleeding arises from cuff and adjacent pedicles. It may be wise to leave a suction drain for few days.

TECHNICAL DIFFICULTIES

It is always a more difficult procedure than cesarean section. Greater downward displacement of bladder is required for cesarean total hysterectomy than for cesarean section. In emergency room therefore it is easy and safer to perform subtotal hysterectomy especially when it is a life saving procedure and when cervix is already filly dilated. At term all tissues around cervix and vagina are lax and the ureters have to be displaced more than in routine cesarean section and clamps should be carefully applied close to uterus to avoid their damage. Due to lax tissues uterus is pulled up surprisingly easily and one may misjudge the level of demarcation between the cervix and vagina and cut the vagina quite low. This may leave a short vagina and future coital problems. Bleeding during hysterectomy in these circumstances is greater; tissue planes are more widely open and risk of deep vein thrombosis should be kept in mind. These difficulties are increased if the patient has undergone one or more cesarean sections previously and this is generally the case in patients under consideration for cesarean hysterectomy. If the placenta is in lower segment or the area is scarred with previous surgery there is an increased incidence of urinary tract injuries. Barclay reported 689 cases of cesarean hysterectomy and described 35 cases of bladder injury, which were recognized at surgery and repaired.[5] Five cases were not recognized and a fistula developed. Two cases of ureteric injury of which only one was recognized intra-operatively. Three cases of bowel injury were also seen. The mesentery of the pelvic colon is closely applied to the left infundibulopelvic ligament and so is liable to injury if left appendages are removed.

COMPLICATIONS

The problems of febrile morbidity, intraoperative hypotension, shock and disseminated intravascular coagulation can be encountered. If appropriate steps are not taken patient can go into multiorgan system failure. The risk of deep vein thrombosis should be considered and when appropriate prophylactic administration of low dose heparin should be given. Injury to adjacent organs like bladder and bowel can take place and if unrecognized intraoperatively, can cause fistula formation in post-operative period. Late complications include Sheehan's syndrome, post-transfusion hepatitis, and hematoma, wound infection, and scar dehiscence and incisional hernia.

ALTERNATIVES TO HYSTERECTOMY

Bilateral internal iliac ligation can be done in patients with uncontrollable postpartum hemorrhage. Knowledge of pelvic anatomy and confidence to do this in emergency situations are prerequisites for surgeons to attempt this method to control bleeding. The *B-Lynch suturing technique* (brace suture) may be useful because of its simplicity of application, life saving potential, relative safety, and its capacity for preserving the uterus and thus fertility. Satisfactory hemostasis can be assessed immediately after application. If it fails, other more radical surgical methods can be used. These should be taught to junior doctors in an attempt to decrease the number of patients transferred in tertiary referral centers for intractable PPH. This will also decrease the number of hysterectomies in intractable PPH. These procedures obviate high-risk surgery and allow maintenance of reproductive ability.

Uterine artery embolization is a superior first-line alternative to surgery for control of obstetric hemorrhage and is a safe and effective alternative to hysterectomy. But this requires technical support and expertise. It is indicated in hemodynamically stable patients with birth canal trauma or uterine atony and clotting anomalies. Use of transcatheter occlusion balloons before embolization allows timely control of bleeding and permits complete embolization of the uterine arteries. Given the improved ultrasonography techniques, diagnosis of some potential high-risk conditions for postpartum hemorrhage, such as placenta previa or accreta, can be made prenatally. The patient can then be prepared with prophylactic placement of arterial catheters, and rapid occlusion of these vessels can be achieved if necessary.

CONCLUSION

Emergency postpartum hysterectomy is associated with significant blood loss, need for transfusion, postoperative complications and longer hospitalization. The combination of prior cesarean section and current placenta previa should alert the obstetrician that emergency postpartum hysterectomy or other newer methods to control post partum bleeding may be needed and the surgeon must be prepared. This procedure is more difficult than a repeat cesarean section. The surgeon must be skillful and anesthesia must be of high order. Postpartum hysterectomy is a necessary life-saving operation. Although maternal mortality is rare, morbidity remains high. Prevention of complications that give rise to hysterectomy and optimally timed surgery should decrease maternal morbidity and mortality.

REFERENCES

1. Speert H. Obstetrics and Gynecology I America: A history. Washington DC: ACOG, 1980.
2. Porro. Dell Amputazione Utero-overica come Complemento di Taglio Caesario. Milan 1876.

3. Suchartwatnachai C, Linasmita V, Chaturachinda K. Obstetric hysterectomy: Ramathibodi's experience 1969-1987. Int J Gynaecol Obstet 1991;36(3):183-6.

4. Yamamoto H, Sagae S, Nishikawa S, Kudo R. Emergency postpartum hysterectomy in obstetric practice. J Obstet Gynaecol Res 2000;26(5):341-5.

5. Barclay DL. Cesarean hysterectomy. Obstet Gynecol NY 35,120-31.

CHAPTER 9

Subtotal Hysterectomy

The technique of a subtotal abdominal hysterectomy is identical to that of Dutta's new technique for a total abdominal hysterectomy until ligation of the uterine arteries has been performed. Following ligation of the uterine arteries, the corpus is amputated. The level of this amputation should always be below the internal cervical os in order to avoid bothersome cyclic menstrual bleeding from remnants of endometrium. It is well to make a V-shaped cut in the cervical stroma and endocervix. This facilitates the closure of the stump and ensures that the endometrium has been removed as well as much of the endocervical canal. The cervical stump is then closed, using figure-of eight sutures of No. 0 delayed-absorbable suture. The clamps on the lateral vaginal angles are replaced by No. 0 delayed-absorbable transfixion sutures. A No. 2-0 delayed-absorbable continuous locking suture is placed around the vaginal margin. Again, the bladder must completely mobilized and retracted inferiorly. An alternative method, closing the vaginal is illustrated. A cutting needle may facilitate placement of this suture, although it is usually not necessary. The cervical stump is suspended by suturing the various ligaments to it as described for a total hysterectomy when the adnexa on both sides have been saved. The suture is first placed through the anterior surface of the cervix. It then picks up the anterior peritoneum and the round ligament. A bite or two is taken in the peritoneum between the round ligament and the tube. The tube to which the ovarian ligament has been tied is next included. One or two bites are taken in the posterior leaf of the broad ligament. In picking up the broad ligament, one should be careful to include only the kinking or ligating the ureter with the suture if wide bites are taken. Finally, a bite is taken in the posterior surface of the cervix. An assistant grasps the ends of the round ligament and the tube and the suspension suture is tied over them. This suture not only suspends the cervix, but also partially peritonizes the pelvis.

If the adnexa have been removed, the suspension and the peritonization are done somewhat differently. The infundibulopelvic ligament may be sufficiently mobile to be brought down to the cervix without tension, but often it is not. In such cases, the leaves of the tip of the broad ligament may be closed separately with a continuous No. 3-0 delayed-absorbable suture as previously described and the stump of the infundibulopelvic ligament buried beneath the peritoneum by a purse-string suture.

A. The uterus has been removed by the open technique, with straight Ochsner clamps being placed on the anterior, lateral, and posterior vaginal margins. Figure-of-eight sutures are placed in each angle of the vagina and carefully tied behind the clamps to secure the vaginal vessels.

B. The vaginal vault is closed with figure-of-eight sutures, the last sutures placed in the midline for traction.

Taking care to avoid the ureters, No. 0 delayed-absorbable suture is passed through both uterosacral ligaments and the posterior vaginal cervix.

Further suspension and reperitonization of the pelvis is accomplished by a continuous No. 0 delayed-absorbable suture that includes the anterior vagina, the cardinal ligament, the anterior edge of broad ligament peritoneum, the round ligament, the utero-ovarian or infundibulopelvic ligament, the posterior edge of broad ligament peritoneum, the uterosacral ligament, and the posterior vagina. A similar suture is placed on the opposite side. And the tubes are covered, it is often desirable to pick up the structures at the angles of the vagina with the suture to cause them to invert beneath the peritoneum.

CHAPTER 10

Total Abdominal Hysterectomy (Modified Richardson's for Benign Tumor)

The technique if abdominal hysterectomy presented here was originally described by Richardson in 1929.

The patient should be properly prepared for operation. After satisfactory general anesthesia is obtained an indwelling urethral catheter is placed in the bladder and left in for continuous bladder drainage. A careful pelvic examination under anesthesia, including a bimanual rectovaginal abdominal examination, is always performed.

To facilitate the operative procedure and to avoid injury to vital structures, adequate exposure through a lower abdominal incision is mandatory. In cases of benign disease, however, the lower abdominal transverse Maylard incision may be preferred. The exposure with a true or modified Pfannenstiel's incision is usually not adequate for the performance of abdominal hysterectomy.

After the incision is made, the upper abdomen is explored. The right kidney, liver, gallbladder, pancreas, stomach, left kidney, and para-aortic lymph nodes are palpated in sequence, and abnormalities are noted. Some type of self-retaining retractor is inserted to expose the pelvic contents. The O'Connor-O'Sullivan or Balfour self-retaining retractors may be used.

Adhesions must be released before the intestines can be placed in the upper abdomen and held there with packs. Restoration of pelvic anatomy by release of adhesions will facilitate the operative procedure.

At this point in the procedure, one should pause and make an assessment of the nature and extent of pelvic pathology; of the anatomical relationships, with particualar reference to the ureters, bladder and rectum; and of the operative procedure to be performed.

The ligament is clamped, ligated with a transfixion suture, and cut. The broad ligament is opened. The anterior leaf of the broad ligament is incised to the point where the bladder peritoneum is reflected onto the anterior lower uterine isthmus in the midline. To avoid unnecessary blood loss, the bladder is not dissected away from the uterus at this point. Two fingers push the posterior leaf of the broad ligament for ward. An incision is made to develop a window in the broad ligament.

If the tube and ovary are to be conserved, three Ochsner clamps are placed across the tube and utero-ovrian ligament as close to the uterus as possible. An incision is made between the middle and the medial clamp. The lateral clamp is replaced with a free tie that completely surrounds the pedicle and occludes the vessels. The middle clamp is replaced by a transfixion suture ligature that is tied securely around both sides of the pedicle.

Clamping, cutting and ligating of the round ligament, the uterine end of the tube, and ovarian ligament or of the infundibulopelvic ligament are carried out in the same manner on the opposite side. The midline reflection of the bladder peritoneum onto the uterus is then freed by extending the incision in the anterior leaf of the broad ligament. If the tube and ovary are to be removed, three Ochsner clamps are placed across the infundibulopelvic ligament, using the window in the broad ligament. After the ureter is located, the lateral-most clamp is placed first. The ligament is incised at the dotted line, and the pedicle is doubly ligated with No. 0 delayed-absorbable suture.

The posterior leaf of the broad ligament is cut on either side parallel with the lateral side of the uterus down to the point of origin of the uterosacral ligaments behind the cervix. Incising the anterior and posterior broad ligament peritoneum will allow the uterine vessels to be exposed and skeletonized before they are clamped. Before clamping and cutting the uterine vessels, the bladder must be mobilized inferiorly by sharp dissection away from the cervix. In order to avoid unnecessary bleeding, this step may be stages as necessary. The posterior leaf of the broad ligament is incised down to the point where the uterosacral ligaments join the cervix, as illustrated dissection across the back of the cervix can be delayed until later to avoid unnecessary bleeding.

After the uterine vessels are skeletonized, they are triply clamped and cut along the dotted lines. To avoid clamping the ureter, the lowest clamp is placed first, at the level of the internal cervical os and at right angles to the lower uterine isthmus. The lowest two clamps are replaced by No. 0 delayed-absorbable suture ligatures. If a total hysterectomy is to be done, the uteurine vessels are dropped away by placing an Ochsner clamp across the upper cardinal ligament between the uterine vessels and the lower uterine isthmus. The tissue is cut and ligated. A flap of peritoneum is dissected from the cervix posteriorly. This will allow the uterosacral ligaments to be isolated and the rectovaginal space to be entered behind the cervix. The uterosacral ligaments are clamped, cut and ligated adjacent to the cervix. Each clamp is replaced by a No. 0 delayed-absorbable suture. A sagittal view showing the bladder dissection completed and indicating depth and direction of the posterior dissection into the rectovaginal space. A sagittal view showing depth and direction of the vesicocervicovaginal dissection. This step serves to displace the bladder and the ureters still further away from the danger zone. Testing the depth of the anterior and posterior dissections. The inset shows the method of segregating the vascular plexus on each side into a narrow zone adjacent to the basal segment of the broad ligament. A T-shaped or V-shaped incision is made in the pubovesicocervical fascia anterior to the cervix. Straight Ochsner clamps are placed across the cardinal ligaments lateral to the cervix and inside the fascia in such a way that the fascia is actually peeled off the cervix. An incision is made at the dotted line and the clamp is replaced with a No. 0 delayed-absorbable suture. Several bites may be needed in each cardinal ligament. After one determines with certainty that the bladder and rectum have been completely dissected away from the vagina curved Ochsner clamps are placed across the vaginal angles and the uterus is removed by incision the vagina below the cervix. Vaginal vault is repaired by running or continuous mattress suture. Peritonization is done with anterior and posterior fasia.

CHAPTER 11

Radical Abdominal Hysterectomy for Invasive Cancer

SURGICAL TREATMENT OF INVASIVE CERVICAL CARCINOMA

To avoid the problems associated with irradiation therapy particulars in young women desiring preservation of ovarian function – a radical Wertheim hystecrectomy and pelvic lymphadenectomy are used for patients with Stage Ib or Stage IIa cervical carcinoma.

In preparation for this procedure, patients require adequate bowel preparation, adequate hydration and adequate blood volume.

A bowel preparation with purgatives and antibiotics is needed mainly when a radical procedure is used for redioresistant carcinoma, because in such cases the operation is usually more extensive and occasionally results in bowel injury. A liquid diet should be provided before surgery to promote complete emptying of the intestinal tract. If bowel resection is planned, a long intestinal tube (Cantor tube) is positional in the ileum on the day before surgery.

Most of the preoperative studies require tasting or enema, so there is a tendency for the patient to become dehydrated. Dehydration is exaggerated by diarrhea produced during the extensive diagnostic studies, including intravenous pyelogram and barium enema. To provide adequate tissue hydration 2 liters of 5% glucose in normal saline are given on the day prior to surgery, and additional intravenous fluid is given until the urinary specific gravity or plasma osmolality is within the normal range.

Blood volume studies are useful initially in evaluating red-cell mass and plasma volume but are not practical for monitoring blood replacement. Hematocrit values and plasma osmolality can be used to accurately evaluate intravascular volume and red cell mass, both before and after surgery. Preoperative transfusion is required until a hematocrit of 40% is achieved.

The placement of a central venous catheter is considered essential for proper monitoring of the patient's intravascular compartment and cardiac reserve during and after radical surgery. Patients with cardiovascular or pulmonary disease that does not preclude radical surgery should have a Swan Ganz catheter inserted into the pulmonary artery before surgery for accurate monitoring of cardiac and pulmonary function (See Chapters 5 and 6). The catheter should not be maintained with a slow infusion, but it should not be used for intravenous fluid replacement. Baseline electrolyte studies, serum protein with albumin-globulin ratio, serum creatinine, and baseline liver function studies are also part of the normal laboratory evaluation of the patient.

RADICAL WERTHEIM HYSTERECTOMY

The classical Wertheim hysterectomy consists of wide resection of the parametrium, dessection of the terminal ureter from the "web" (vesicouterine ligament), wide resection of the ureterosacral ligaments, and removal of the upper 3 to 4 cm of the vagina and paravaginal tissues, along with a thorough pelvic lymphadenectomy.

Following proper abdominal and vaginal preparation, an indwelling catheter is placed in the bladder to keep it decompressed throughout the operative procedure. A low midline incision, extending from approximately 3 cm abovel the umbilicus to the symphysis pubis, is required for adequate exposure.

  1. *Abdominal and pelvic exploration:* The intra-abdominal and pelvic viscera, the retroperitoneal lymph nodes,

and the parietal and visceral surfaces of the peritoneal cavity must be evaluated for possible metastatic tumor. The liver surface, both hemidiaphragms, the mesentery of the large and small bowel, and the serosal surfaces of the bowel should be palpated retroperitoneally to check for possible gross abnormalities.

2. Of paramount importance is the evaluation of the para-aortic lymph node chain. The para-aortic area must be carefully palpated from the region of the bifurcation of the aorta to the celiac plexus.

3. If the lower nodes below the inferior mesenteric artery and vein appear to be normal and are proven histologically by frozen-section study to be negative for metastatic tumor, the patient can be assumed with relative certainty not to have metastases higher up the lymphatic chain. Histologic proof is essential, since 15% of para-aortic node metastases are occult and occur in normal-appearing, soft luymph nodes.

4. The pelvic lymph node dissection can be extended routinely to include the lower 3 to 4 cm of the aorta and vena cava. Extrapelvic nodes are studied separately by frozen section before the hysterectomy is started. Histologic findings from extrapelvic nodes are particularly important in high-risk cases associated with one or more factors indicating a poor prognosis.

5. Evaluation of any extension of the pelvic tumor is carried out by examining the course of the lymphatic drainage and carefully palpating all the pelvic vessels.

6. The paravesical and pararectal spaces are important anatomical landmarks because the intervening base of the broad ligament can be explored between these

areas. When evidence of extracervical disease is detected in the broad ligament or at the lateral pelvic wall, the surgical procedure should be abandoned and the patient treated with full pelvic irradiation.

7. Radical Wertheimn hysterectomy. Opening the anterior leaf of the broad ligament after ligating the round ligament and infundibulopelvic ligament.

8. Developing the paravesical space to the region of the pelvic floor.

9. Radical Wertheim hysterectomy (Continued). Opening the posterior leal of the broad ligament for development of the pararectal fossa. Paravesical and pararectal fossae with intervening base of broad ligament attached to the pelvic floor and lateral pelvic wall.

10. Pelvic lymphadenectomy with dissection of the right common iliac vessels and their brances, including the external iliac and hypogastric artery and vein. Note the attachment of the ureter to the parietal peritoneum. The genitofemoral nerve courses along the psoas muscle.

11. Entry into obturator space by medial reflection of the external iliac vessels.

12. Dissection of the obturator fossa showing the obturator nerve with areolar tissue attached superiorly to the external iliac vessels.

13. Metzenbaum scissors inserted above the ureter in the "web" or ureteral tunnel of the broad ligament. Note the ligated uterine artery in the anterior fascial sheath of the tunnel. The roof of the tunnel is opened between clamps, with the ureter attached to the posterior sheath.

14. Excision of the posterior sheath of the vesicouterine ligament. Note the incision line along the medial border of the terminal ureter.

15. Clamping and incision of the lateral portion of the cardinal ligament adjacent to the lateral pelvic wall. (B) Excised ligament showing the pelvic floor and levator muscles. The dissected obturator nerve is seen in the obturator space.

16. Cutting the cul-de-sac peritoneum as it reflects onto the rectum. Ureters course laterally devoid of peritoneum. Dissection of the rectovaginal septum with development of the rectal stalks (uterosacral ligaments) laterally. Clamping of the rectal stalks, including the uterosacral ligament. The ureter is gently retracted to avoid trauma.

17. Dissection of the bladder from the vagina and excision of the paravaginal fascia from the lateral pelvic wall. The lower ureter is retracted from the operating field.

18. Opening the vagina and securing the lower vaginal cuff. The upper 2 to 3 cm of vagina are included with the surgical specimen.

19. Open vaginal cuff with continuous locking suture for homeostasis. The ureters are seen laterally and the denuded rectum posteriorly.

POSTOPERATIVE COMPLICATIONS FOLLOWING A RADICAL WERTHEIM HYSTERCTOMY

Bladder Complications

1. *Fistula:* The posterior bladder wall may be lacerated or torn during the extensive dissection of the bladder base from the cervix and upper vagina. This injury not be grossly visible and should routinely be checked for the completion of the procedure by water cystoscopy or by distending the bladder with chromogen-colored

saline. Suturing the bladder peritoneum to the margins of the anterior vaginal wall protects the bladder and terminal urters from secondary infection and subsequent fistula formation. Suprapublic bladder drainage for 2 to 4 weeks postoperatively maintains the bladder and terminal ureters at rest until adequate collateral circulation has been established.

2. *Neurogenic bladder dysfunction:* Both motero and sensory neurogenic bladder dysfunction are common complications of radical dissection of the base of the broad ligament. Both sympathetic and para sympathetic nerve fibers are contained in the pelvic nerve plexus and interruption of these nerve fibers during surgery produces the problem. A beneficial effect on bladder function when the pars nervosa (posterior) portion of the cardinal ligament is preserved. Preservation of the lateral mesentery of the terminal ureter at the ureterovesical junction was found to improve both the sensory and the motor function of the bladder.

Ureteral Complications

Fistula and stenosis: Devascularization and ischemic necrosis of the wall of the terminal ureter have proven to be the more serous complications or the radical Wertheim procedure. The ureter is watched meticlulously during the entire surgical process to prevent vascular trauma or injury to the muscularis. These is reduced the incidence of ureteral fistula to less than 2%.

Pelvic Lymphocyst

The accumulation of lymph within the pelvis from retrograde lymphatic drainage was previously noted to be a common complication of the radical hysterectomy with lymphadenctomy.

Pelvic Cellulitis

Adequate vaginal and abdominal drainage of the operative site greatly diminished the incidence of pelvic celluslitis following radical pelvic surgery. The use of prophylactic antibiotics has markedly reduced the incidence of pelvic cellulites to less than 5% of all cases.

Venous Thrombosis and Pulmonary Embolus

Venous thrombosis: The patient who undergoes redical pelvic surgery has a higher risk of developing venous thrombosis of the lower extremity than patients who have other types of gynecologic surgery.

Prolonged immobilization of the lower extremities during the lengthy operative procedure is a major cause of intraoperative venous stasis and clot formation. At least 50% of the patients with this complication develop it during the surgical procedure.

Heparin, in a dose of 5,000 units given subcutaneously three times daily, beginning 2 hours before surgery and every 8 hours thereafter for 5 days, has decreased the incidence of thrombosis.

Pulmonary embolus: Clinical evidence collected through ^{125}I fibrinogen scans indicates that approximately 3 to 5% of patients with occult venous thrombosis of the lower extremities will develop a pulmonary embolus.

The day after surgery, 100 microcuries of ^{125}I-labeled fibrinogen should be injected and daily monitoring should be initiated. Rarely does a pulmonary embolus occur after full anticoagulation has been achieved. In such cases, further migration of the venous clot must be stopped either by ligating the inferior vena cava or by using an intracaval Silastic umbrella.

HEMORRHAGE

Intraoperative bleeding: Most problems with bleeding occur with the dissection of the cardinal ligament and the hypogastric vessels. Only meticulous dissection of the pelvic floor can prevent bleeding complications. When venous bleeding does occur, the laceration site may be difficult to identify. Bleeding from an indefinite source can be stopped by compressing the pelvic floor veins with either a sponge stick or an abdominal pack held firmly against the entire area for no less than 7 minutes. Dissection should not proceed until full control of the bleeding has been established.

The most serious problem for hemostasis occurs when the wall of a major pelvic vein has been severely traumatized and retracts out of the operative field. Hemorrhage from a deep pelvic vein can rarely be controlled by ligating the hypogastric artery because the lower extremities and vena cava provide extensive collateral venous circulation.

More extensive damage to the wall of the external iliac or hypogastric vein must be repaired by first placing vascular clamps above and below the area of injury and then suturing the defect.

Postoperative Hemorrhage

Since all of the blood supply to the pelvis is skeletonized as part of the radical Wertheim procedure, hemorrhage can only result from bleeding that was not completely controlled during surgery. To control bleeding postoperatively, the pelvis may be packed with a multiple gauze tamponade that is extended ring (Logothetopulostic back). Pelvis packs should be advanced within 24 to 48 hours and removed shortly thereafter to prevent infection from ascending bacteria.

Modificaiton of the Radical Wertheim Hysterectomy

The modifiedWertheim hysterectomy it was initially used for the treatment of carcinoma *in situ*, and more recently was designed for the treatment of moicroinvasive carcinoma. Whereas the radical Wertheim procedure removes the medial one-third to one-half of (TELINDE) the cardinal ligament but does not remove the pelvic lymph nodes. As a result, the ureter is less subject to tauma, since the dissection is confined pelvic ureters and the terminal ureter is not dissected from the web. Now that colposcopy and conization are used to make a more precise diagnosis of in situ and microinvasive carcinoma, the modified Wertheim hysterectomy has a more limited use.

Rutledge uses a similar modified radical hysterectomy by displacing the ureters widely, but not dissecting them from their fascial beds, and removing the proximal one-third to one-half of the parametrium along with a wide vaginal cuff. This type of radial hysterectomy, combined with a pelvic lymphadenectomym is the operation performed today in many clinics, since the operation performed today in many clinics, since the ultraradical treatment of the cardinal ligament had done little to improve the survival rate. Removing the lateral half of the broad ligament appears to do little more than to strip the blood and nerve supply from the lower ureter and base of the bladder.

The modified Wertheim may also be used for bulky endocervical barrel-shaped tumors, both squamous and adenocarcinomatous, that require hysterectomy after full pelvic and intracavitary irradiation. In such cases, pelvic lymphadenectomy is not done. In order to remove the microlymphatics and tumor emboli that are associated with central recurrence of bulky lesions, a good margin of parasection tissue should be removed. More radical dissection is not warranted, however, and usually results in a high incidence of fistula of the blader, ureters, and rectum, because megavoltage irradiation must be used.

CHAPTER 12

Abdominal Hysterectomy for Difficult Cases

FIBROID

Broad Ligament Fibroid

In true broad ligament fibroid since the fibroid arises from lateral wall of uterus, hence ureter is situated lateral to the fibroid whereas in false broad ligament fibroid ureter is situated medial to the tumor. Hence, every care to be taken not to injure ureter, rectum, sigmoid colon and cecum.

Cervical Fibroid

To remove lateral cervical fibroid and posterior cervical fibroid appears to be more difficult than that of central and anterior cervical fibroid. Hence, here problem is injury to the ureter and uterine artery. Therefore every care is to be taken to ligate the uterine artery and descending cervical artery after taking adequate care to the ureter and bladder.

Big Posterior Fibroid

To remove this tumor fingers to be inserted in between capsule and fibroid. Once fibroid is removed. Uterine artery (B) is ligated first to be followed by Abdominal Hysterectomy. Here care is to be taken not to injure – small intestine, rectum, sigmoid colon and ureter.

OVARIAN CYST (BIG)

To remove ovarian cyst – First step is to ligate (Twice) the infundibulopelvic ligament to be followed by removing of ovarian tumor by cutting the infundibulopelvic ligament then proceed for abdominal hysterectomy. Here care to be taken not to injure ureter, sigmoid colon and rectum and cecum.

ENDOMETRIOSIS

In severe endometriosis (frozen pelvis) – Subtotal Hysterectomy is usually performed because of anatomical difficulty. So every care is to be taken not to injure the bladder, ureter and intestines. Big Chocolate cyst (ovarian) – after opening the cyst – blood is to be drained from the cyst for reducing the size of the tumor from cyst – identify the infundibulopelvic ligament and then ligate and cut the structures in infundibulopelvic ligament followed by ligation of uterine artery – proceed for subtotal hysterectomy. Screening of cervical pathology is to be done during postoperative check-up. Sometimes it is very difficult to identify the structures hence urosurgeon, vascular surgeon and general surgeon may require during operation.

SEVERE PELVIC INFLAMMATORY DISEASES

Due to dense adhesion it is very difficult to identify structures hence same procedure to be followed as that of endometriosis. Precaution to be taken not to injure ureter, bladder and intestine.

CHAPTER 13

Complications and Management Following Abdominal Hysterectomy Operation

Serious morbidity and occasional mortality still occur from abdominal hysterectomy. Abdominal hysterectomy places the urinary tract and intestinal tract at greater risk of injury and also involves making an incision in the abdominal wall. Vaginal hysterectomy, on the other hand, is often associated with anterior and posterior colporrhaphy. Although the complications of vaginal and abdominal hysterectomy are often compared the operations are not comparable and are not done for comparable pathology such as injuries to the urinary tract. Reperitonizaiton is completed with a continuous No. 3-0 delayed-absorbable suture that approximates the edge of the bladder peritoneum to the edge of the cul-de-sac peritoneum. The ovaries should be left laterally.

MORTALITY

Of 1283 women who underwent abdominal hysterectomy in the 1982 study by Dicker and associates, only one died postoperatively. She had a deep venous thrombosis and died of complications of venography. Of 4283 abdominal hysterectomies for benign disease reported by Amirikia and Evans, seven preventable postoperative deaths occurred (0.16%), including three from pulmonary embolus, two from infection, and one from postoperative shock and pulmonary edema. White reports a large series in which the incidence of operative death after hysterectomy was 0.7%. The major causes of postoperative death today include cardiac arrest, pulmonary embolus, and sepsis, with occasional cases of postoperative hemorrhage, intestinal obstrauction, and subarachnoid hemorrhage.

OPERATIVE AND POSTOPERATIVE HEMORRHAGE

The most common serious post-hysterectomy complication is bleeding. This incidence is high. Intraperitoneal hemorrhage, which is occult, is far more dangerous, since its detection may be delayed. On the other hand, when pedicles are covered with peritoneum and the vaginal cuff is left open, postoperative bleeding may be more apparent coming through the vagina. Although it is easier to control intraoperative hemorrhage during an abdominal than during a vaginal hysterectomy, most of the bleeding occurs postoperatively and is usually related either to faulty surgical technique or to technical difficulties during the ligation of the vascular pedicles of the broad ligament. When profuse bleeding does occur, it may start suddenly and assume alarming proportions in a remarkably short time so that quick action is imperative. It can not be assumed that the patient who spends a few hours in the recovery room without evidence of bleeding or hypo-tension is secure from the risk of postoperative hemorrhage. If there is a small unsecured vessel bleeding into the peritoneal cavity, the occult hemorrhage may not produce clinical signs of hypovolemia for several hours. Patients must be observed closely for at least 24 hours post-operatively. Postoperative hematocrits should be obtained routinely when the operation is completed, on the morning of the first postoperative day, and at any other time when there is the slightest suggestion of intraperitoneal bleeding or hypovolemia.

Bleeding that occurs directly after the operation is usually due to improper suturing of the angles of the vaginal cuff and should be attended to immediately by returning the patient to the operating room and suturing the cuff per vaginum. Such bleeding is usually transvaginal and evident immediately. However, some may be intra-abdominal, especially if the peritoneum has not been securely closed over the pedicles. In connection with this complication, it is important to re-emphasize the rationale of the closure of the angles of the vagina. To ensure adequate ligation of the vaginal arteries and veins that arise from the hypogastric vessels, the vaginal angle suture must be placed following abdominal hysterectomy so that the free ends of the ligature are tied around the lateral margin of the vaginal cuff. Techniques for securing the vaginal angle are one of these techniques of anatomical closure of the vascular angles of the vagina is used, it is unusual to have postoperative bleeding after a total abdominal hysterectomy. Post-hysterectomy bleeding most frequently occurs from the seventh to the fourteenth postoperative day. At this time, catgut sutures may partially dissolve and lose their tensile strength. Also, edematous vaginal tissue may slough and separate and cut through tightly tied suture material that this type of bleeding is quite unavoidable and will occur regardless of the method of closure of the vaginal vault.

OPERATIVE INJURIES OF THE URETER

Injury to the pelvic ureter is one of the most serious operative complications of gynecologic surgery. Occurring on the average in between 0.1% and 1.5% of all cases of major pelvic surgery. This type of injury is associated with high morbidity, ureterovaginal fistulas, and the potential loss of kidney function.

Type of Injury and Operative Procedure

Operative injury to the ureter results from one of four type of trauma: ligation, crushing, transection, or angulation with secondary obstruction. Each type of injury may be either partial or complete. Two-thirds of ureteral injuries result from an abdominal hysterectomy as compared to one-third that occur as a complication of a vaginal hysterectomy. Ureteral injury usually occurs in one of four strategic anatomical locations. In the cardinal ligament where the ureter psses beneath the uterine vessels: beyond the uterine artery where the ureter lies adjacent to the anterior vaginal wall and enters the base of the bladder; at or below the infundibulopelvic ligament; and less frequently, along the course of the broad ligament, including the uterosacral. Of the four common sites of ureteral injury, the first is the most frequent. If the uterine vessels are clamped carefully close to the uterus, with the clamps at right angles to the internal cervical os and within the pubovesicocervical fascia, the danger of ureteral injury is reduced significantly. The danger of injury is reduced significantly. The danger of injury to the ureter is greatest in cases in which the vessels slip from the clamp or the ligature and reclamping is attempted quickly in the presence of profuse bleeding.

The second most common injury occurs in the distal, terminal 3 to 4 cm of the ureter between the uterine artery and the trigone of the bladder. In a difficult pelvic dissection where the bladder base and adjacent ureter have not been displaced adequately from the upper vagina and base of the cardinal ligament, the paracervical and paravaginal clamps or sutures may inadvertently crush or ligate the ureter as it passes medially to enter the bladder.

The third common site of ureteral injury is at the pelvic brim. A short infundibulopelvic ligament may result from distortion of the normal anatomy by a variety of disease processes, such as a large ovarian tumor, a paraovarian cyst, pelvic endometriosis, or a large tubo-ovarian abscess. The clamp placed on the ovarian vessels in such cases may include the underlying rueter unless this is carefully identified. Prior to clamping the infundibulopelvic ligament, it is incumbent upon the surgeon to identify the location of the ureter as it enters the pelvis and to make certain that the pedicle clamp does not encroach upon the underlying ureter. If necessary, the location of this segment of the ureter should be verified by opening the peritoneum lateral to the bifurcation of the common iliac artery and reflecting the peritoneum medially until the ureter comes into full view. With this anatomical security, the distorted ovarian pedicle can be clamped safely without risk of injury to the adjacent ureter.

With large pelvic tumors, especially those that have developed between the leaves of the broad ligament, freeing the tumor from the pelvis may endanger an adherent ureter. Although the broad ligament is the least common site of ureteral injury, identification and exposure of the pelvic ureter may be necessary. When ureteral identfication is desirable during the operation, it is important to locate the ureter at the pelvic brim, open the peritoneum on the lateral side of the ureter, and leave the pelvic peritoneum and the periureteral tissue attached to the ureter, for in this tissue lie the important blood vessels that supply the ureter.

When an intraligamentary fibroid, an adherent ovarian tumor, or advanced pelvic inflammatory disease suggests proximity or adherence of the disease to the pelvic wall, preoperative catheterization of the ureter(s) is both time saving and a great safety factor. By this procedure, the ureter can be identified more easily and speedily during the operation and its course can be followed throughout the pelvis without dissection and without the attendant danger of impairment of its blood supply. In the event that a catheter has not been inserted preoperatively and the broad ligament anatomy is distorted by extensive inflammation, dense adhesions from endometriosis, or other obscuring disease, the bladder dome may be opened and a catheter inserted into the ureter through the ureteral orifice. Alternatively, the ureter can be identified as it crosses the common iliac artery to enter the pelvis, the peritoneum can be opened on the lateral side, and the entire pelvic ureter can be exposed to the base of the broad ligament. The ability to skillfully trace the course of the pelvic ureter, without separating ardizing its blood supply, should be within the surgical capability and experience of every gynecologic surgeon.

A gynecologic surgeon to become "ureter conscious" and to develop a routine method of ensuring the integrity of both ureters before concluding a major operative procedure. Whether direct palpation, mobilization and inspection, ureteral catheterization, or some other means of ureteral identification, the surgeon should develop some fail-safe method of evaluating the intergrity of the pelvic ureter at the time of the operative procedure. An intravenous chromogen test has proven to be an effective method of providing this assurance. Prior to closing the peritoneal cavity, either abdominally or vaginally, the surgeon may quickly ascertain bilateral ureteral integrity by inspecting the ureteral orifices in the bladder trigone with a cystoscope or hysteroscope after an intravenous bolus of 5 cc of indigo carmine or methylene blue dye has been injected. If both ureters are intact, the ureteral or ifices will spurt a blue-colored urine with equal pressure and frequency. This simple procedure does not require urologic consultation or special expertise in cystoscopic procedures. Any endoscopic instrument may be used if a cystoscope is not readily available, including a laparoscope or hystero-scope. Should a ureteral orifice fail to spurt dye after the patient has been adequately hydrated, the ureter should be explored along its entire pelvic course to determine if injury has occurred. It is important to keep in mind the timeless statement that has benefited many noted pelvic surgeons: It is no sin to injure the ureter during pelvic surgery, but it is a serious sin to fail to recognize it.

POSTOPERATIVE INFECTION

Major infections include pelvic cellulities, infected hematoma or abscess above the vaginal cuff, abdominal wound infection, and adnexal infections. Diagnosis is made by finding tenderness and induration or a mass on palpation of the affected area in a febrile postoperative patient who complains of increasing lower abdominal pain. Gently probing the vaginal cuff or abdominal incision may yield pus, which should be cultured for both an-aerobic and aerobic bacteria. Cultures from the vaginal cuff on the abdominal incision of women with major infection after abdominal hysterectomy. Included in the list of aerobic bacteria cultured were the following: *Staphylococcus* (2 species), *Escheichia coli, Enterobacter* (3 species), *Klebsiella pneumoniae,* and *Proteus mirabilis*. The list of anaerobic bacteria included: *Peptostreptococcus* (3 species), *Streptococcus* intermedius, *Peptococcus* magnus, Gaffkya anaerobia, *Clostridium* (5 species), *Bacteroides* (4 species), and *Fusobacterium nucleatum*.

The age of the patient is an important factor that is related to postoperative infections. The highest incidence of postoperative infections. The highest incidence of postoperative infections seems to occurs in women under 40 years of age. Medically indigent patients have a higher rate of postoperative infections. The lack of hemostasis undoubtedly facilitates the growth of bacteria in traumatized tissue. Thrombophlebitis may be associated with postoperative fever.

NECROTIZING FASCITIS

Necrotizing fascitis is a rare postoperative complication of pelvic surgery, usually resulting from an incisional infection that involves the fascia of the anterior abdominal wall. The predominant B-hemolytic *E. coli, Proteus,* and *Pseudomonas, Clostridium welchii.* This complication of pelvic surgery remains as one of the more lethal and difficult clinical problems to control. The morbidity and mortality from necrotizing fascitis remain distressingly high and are directly related to the age of the patient, the presence of associated disease process, and, more important, the time interval from the onset of the infection to the recognition and institution of therapy. Vaginal vault granulation, post-hysterectomy prolapse of the fallopian tube, hematoma or abscess in the vaginal apex are reporated. Late complications following hysterectomy are unusual. The psychological depression and sexual dysfunction and emotional difficulties may be increased after hys-terectomy. Post-hysterectomy prolapse of the vaginal vault is also reporated.

MANAGEMENT OF INJURIES

Several general principles apply to the management and repair of all lower urinary tract injuries. The administration of prophylactic antibiotics should be considered. The extent of the damage to the urinary tract must be explored. Devitalized tissues must be excised. Urinary tract repairs should be performed with small-caliber delayed absorbable (polyglactin or polyglycolic acid) or absorbable (chromic) suture. Absolutely no tension should be placed on the repair site. Extraperitoneal suction drainage should be placed adjacent to, but not in contact with, all retroperitoneal repairs. Bladder drainage is important to reduce tension within the wall of the bladder during the healing phase.

RECOGNITION OF URETERAL INJURY

Ureteral Dye Injection

The integrity of a single ureter can be demonstrated by injecting indigo carmine dye into the lumen of the ureter above the surgical site. Intravenous injection of indigo carmine (slow infusion of 5 ml) normally results in the excretion of blue urine within 5 to 10 minutes. If the dye injection is accompanied by an increase in intravenous fluids or mannitol or the administration of a diuretic, dye excretion may be enhanced. When an intravenous dye, such as indigo carmine, is administered, the passes of blue urine means that at least one renal unit is functioning. To determine which renal unit is functioning, the surgeon must perform either cytoscopy (suprapublic or transurethral) or cystotomy. Leakage of blue urine into the operative field is evidence of lower urinary tract injury. This requires further investigation.

Cystoscopy may performed transurethrally or suprapubically. Transurethral cystoscopy is facilitated by the routine use of universal stirrups. Suprapublic cystoscopy is called telescopy. When telescopy is completed, the cystotomy site may be used for subsequent suprapublic bladder catheter drainage. The intravenous injection of indigo carmine (5 ml) just before cystoscopy enables the examiner to determine ureteric function, as evidenced by the excretion of blue urine. When either ureter fails to excrete blue urine, the reason must be determined.

CYSTOTOMY

A cystotomy is another is another method of observing the inside of the bladder. Ideally, the cystotomy should be placed in the extraperitoneal portion of the dome of the bladder. If intravenous indigo carmine is administered, the excretion of blue urine helps determine the integrity of each renal unit.

URETERAL CATHETERIZATION

Intraoperative ureteral catheterization is usually performed by cystoscopy or cytotomy. It may be also performed by ureterotomy. When cystoscopy or cystotomy is performed, the ureters may be catheterized using a small pediatric feeding tube, ureteral catheter, or ureteral stent. The pediatric feeding tube is more easily passed through the ureteric tunnels. The tube is usually used intraoperatively to demonstrate ureteral patency, but it can be used for short-term postoperative ureteral drainage (Fig. 13.1).

Resistance to the passage of a ureteral catheter suggests kinking or obstruction of the ureter. The drainage of urine through the catheter documents renal function. Catheters and stents may be left in place when there are obstructions, crush injuries, or ureteric repairs to drain urine from the kidneys, help prevent stenosis of the ureter, and facilitate healing.

Intravenous Urography

Intravenous urography may be performed intraoperatively to determine renal function and to document the integrity of the lower urinary tracts.

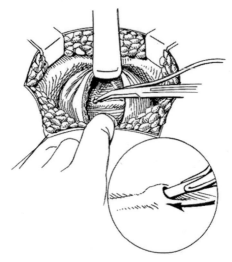

Fig. 13.1: Technique of ureteral catheter passage
after cystomy has been performed

Management of Ureteral Injury

a. Ureteral angulations and kinks should be released if
   they cause significant obstruction.
b. A ligated ureter should have the ligating suture
   removed.
c. Minor ureteral crush injuries may be managed with
   stenting ; singnificant crush injuries require resection
   of the damaged segment and ureteroneocystostomy or
   ureteroureterostomy. Partial lacerations of a ureter can
   be repaired by appropriate placement of several
   absorbable or delayed absorbable sutures. Complete
   lacerations of the ureter and loss of a segment of ureter
   require definitive repair.

The surgical procedures recommended for ureteral
repair vary according to the ureteral segment that is

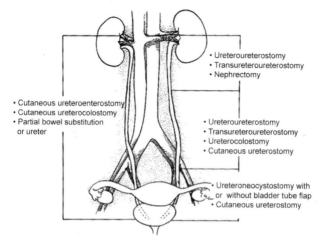

Fig. 13.2: Various techniques of ureter and bladder operation

involved. Because most gynecologic injuries to the ureter involve its distal 4 to 5 cm, most can be repaired by ureteroneocystostomy. Injuries just below the pelvic brim may be repaired by ureteroureterostomy or ureteroneocystostomy. Ureteroneocystotomy is not recommended for injuries above the pelvic brim (Fig. 13.2).

URETERONEOCYSTOSTOMY

Ureteroneocystostomy is the procedure of choice for injuries involving the terminal 4 to 5 cm of either ureter. The distal ureteral segment is ligated with permanent suture at its entry into the bladder. If the proximal ureter has a non-viable segment, this is excised. The end of the ureter is then tagged with a ling through-and-through suture. The bladder may be mobilized by the release of its attachments to the posterior surface of the publis. An extraperitoneal cystotomy is performed in the dome of the bladder, and the base of the bladder is displaced towards the end of the injured ureter. A Kelly's clamp is used to make a direct puncture through the full thickness of the base of the bladder at an appropriate location to allow the tagged distal end of the ureter to be brought into the bladder. When this is accomplished, and at least 1 cm of ureter is inside of the bladder, the end of the ureter is spatulated bilaterally, and its distal flaps are secured to the inside of the bladder with No. 3-0 chromic sutures. The adventitia of the ureter is anchored to the outside of the bladder with several No. 3-0 delayed absorbable sutures. Most importantly, no tension should be placed on the ureter or the bladder at the site of the ureteroneocystostomy. If there is tension on the anastomosis, it should be relieved by a vesicopsoas hitch procedure. If a vesicopsoas hitch is needed, it is best performed before reimplantation or reanastomosis of the ureter (Figs 13.3 and 13.4). Surgeons differ on the need for ureteral stenting following ureteroneocystostomy. If there is any question about the use of a stent, one should be used. The site of the anastomosis should be drained by an extraperitoneal suction drain. The cystotomy should be closed and the bladder should be drained continuously for at least 7 days.

URETEROURETEROSTOMY

The simplest ureteroureterostomy involves the tension-free reanastomosis of two cut ends of a ureter. When there is loss of a ureteral segment, there may be a need for bladder or kidney mobilization, a bladder extension procedure, trans-ureteroureterostomy, or the interposition of an intestinal segment.

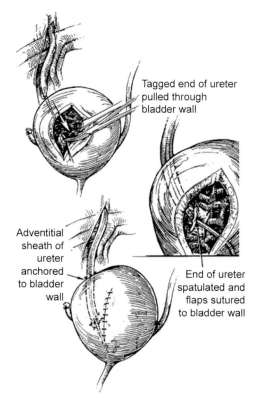

Tagged end of ureter pulled through bladder wall

Adventitial sheath of ureter anchored to bladder wall

End of ureter spatulated and flaps sutured to bladder wall

Fig. 13.3: Ureteroneocystostomy: After the ureter is divided and the listal segment ligated, an incision is made in the bladder wall near the old ureteral orifice, and the tagged end of the ureter is pulled through the bladder wall. The end of the ureter is spatulated, and the flaps are sutured to the bladder mucosa. The adventitial sheath of the ureter is anchored to the bladder wall. (From Hurt WG, Segreti EM. Intraoperative ureteral injuries and urinary diversion. In Nichols DH, Clarke-Pearson D, eds. *Gynecologic and Obstetric Surgery,* 2nd ed. Mosby, St Louis, 1999, with permission)

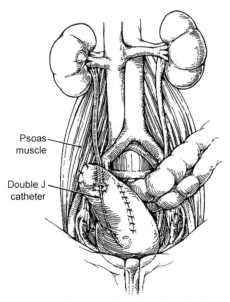

Psoas muscle

Double J catheter

Fig. 13.4: Vesicopsoas hitch operation: Used for distal ureteral injuries in which there is tension on a ureteroneocystostomy or uretero-ureterostomy. This technique brings the bladder cephalad to relieve tension on the suture site. (From Hurt WG Segreti EM. Intraoperative ureteral injuries and urinary diversion. In Nichols DH, Clarke-Pearson D, eds. *Gynecologic and Obstetric Surgery,* 2nd ed. Mosty, St. Louis, 1999, with permission)

In performing a ureteroureterostomy, the viable cut ends of each ureteral segment are spatulated for a distance of about 0.5 cm to help prevent stenosis of the anastomosis. A ureteral catheter is inserted into the ureter to brige the anastomotic site. Four to six interrupted full-thickness No. 4-0 chromic sutures are used to perform the anastomosis. The anastomotic site should be drained by an extraperitoneal suction drain to prevent the accumulation of blood, serum, or urine. This drain should remain in place until the ureteral catheter has been removed. The ureteral catheter should be left in place for at least 7 days. Postoperative bladder drainage is usually recommended.

BLADDER MOBILIZATION AND EXTENSION

When performing a ureteroneocystostomy or uretero-ureterostomy, no tension should be placed on the site of the anastomosis. Dissection of the retropublic space (of Retzius) frees the bladder from its attachments to the posterior symphysis and allows it to be mobilized toward the site of the repair. If this is done and there is still some tension on the anastomosis, the surgeon should consider performing a psoas hitch or bladder extension procedure.

The vesicopsoas hitch is performed by placing one or two fingers through an extraperitoneal cystotomy and pushing the bladder toward the psoas muscle on the side of the anticipated ureteral repair. If dissection of the retropublic space and a psoas hitch do not give enough mobility to the bladder to allow a satisfactory ureteral implantation or reanastomosis, the creation of the bladder flap made into a tubular structure and ureteral implantation should be considered.

Bridging the gap between the cut end of a ureter and the bladder is possible by performing an ileoureteroneocystostomy. A segment of ileum of sufficient length and with adequate blood supply is isolated from the bowel. Its distal end is sutured to a cystostomy site in the dome of the bladder, and the cut end of the ureter is implanted into its proximal end. The continuity of the ileum is then reestablished.

TRANSURETEROURETEROSTOMY

When so much of the ureter has been lost that it is imposible to perform a ureteroneocystostomy or ureteroureterostomy, a transureteroureterostomy should be considered. In performing a transureteroureterostomy, the proximal ureter is mobilized and passed retroperitoneally below the inferior mesenteric artery and in front of the great vessels to meet the opposite ureter. The recipient ureter is longitudinally incised, and an end-to-side anastomosis is performed using full-thickness No. 4-0 absorbable sutures. The anastomosis should be watertight but not ischemic. The anastomotic site should be drained by an extraperitoneal suction drain. Ureteral catheters are not usually necessary.

CUTANEOUS URETEROSTOMY

A cutaneous ureterostomy should not be considered a permanent method of urinary diversion. It may be done when the patient's chances of survival are limited, or in cases in which the surgeon is not prepared to perform a more definite repair. The procedure is performed by bringing out retroperitoneally the cut end of the ureter through the skin and performing a ureteral-skin anastomosis. Ureteral catheters are not usually necessary.

Extraperitoneal suction drains should be placed to the site of, but not in contact with, all internal ureteral anastomoses. These drains should remove all blood, serum, lymph, and urine that collect near the anastomosis. They are not usually removed until all ureteral catheters and stents have been removed.

Continuous bladder catheter drainage, either transurethrally or suprapubically, should be initiated whenever there is a cystotomy, ureteroneocystostomy, or ureteroure-terostomy. In the latter case, when there is no cystotomy, the bladder catheter may be removed before the ureteral catheter or stent is removed.

The repair of ureteric injuries should be followed by an intravenous urogram to determine the integrity of the repair and the presence or absence of a stenosis. This is done to detect fistulas or conditions that might cause kidney damage.

RECOGNITION OF BLADDER INJURY

Bladder Dye Instillations

If surgery is performed with an indigo carmine solution inside the bladder, partial lacerations of the bladder wall reveal the underlying blue mucosa. Penetrations and lacerations of the bladder are indicated by blue dye leaking onto the surgical field.

The integrity of the bladder wall cannot be tested thoroughly until the bladder is filled with 300 to 400 ml of an appropriate liquid-distending medium (sterile water or normal saline containing indigo carmine dye or sterile milk or infant's formula). The bladder can be filled using a single-channel or double-channel transurethral catheter. In difficult cases, repetitive emptying and filling of the bladder is facilitated by the placement of an indwelling three-channel transurethral balloon catheter.

Cystoscopy

Cystoscopy may be performed transurethrally portion of the dome of the bladder, and the inside of the bladder may be examined thoroughly for injuries.

Management of Bladder Injury

Intraoperative repair of bladder injuries varies slightly according to the location of the injury. Extraperitoneal lacerations in the dome of the bladder my be closed with one or two layers of No. 3-0 absorbable or delayed absorbable suture. The suture may be placed in an interrupted or running fashion, depending on the type and extent of the bladder may be used for the insertion of a bladder catheter for postoperative suprapublic bladder drainage.

Transperitoneal laceration of the bladder and lacerations of the base of the bladder should be repaired in two layers, using No. 3-0 absorbabale or delayed-absorbable interrupted or running suture. Also, these lacerations should be covered by a layer of peritoneum or an omental flap (Fig. 13.5). This procedure separates the injury from adjacent structures and cushions the repairs

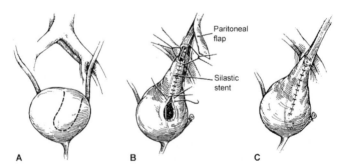

Fig. 13.5: Boari-Ockerblad bladder flap. **A.** Bladder flap is outlined on the bladder. **B.** Bladder flap is created, and ureter is sewn into its end. **C.** Bladderflap and ureteral anastomosis are completed. (From Hurt WG Segreti EM. Intraoperative ureteral injuries and urinary diversion. In Nichols DH, Clarke-Pearson D, (Eds). *Gynecologic and Obstetric Surgery,* 2nd ed. Mosty, St. Louis, 1999, with permission)

by adding bulk. An omental flap brings in new tissue with its own separate blood supply. Significant bladder repairs should have continuous bladder drainage for at least 7 days to facilitate healing.

RECOGNITION OF URETHRAL INJURY

Catheter Insertion

Intraoperatively, urethral injuries are most often diagnosed by the surgeon seeing the catheter through an incision in the wall of the urethra. Small clamps or probes may be used to confirm the injury.

Urethroscopy

Urethroscopy is best performed with a special female urethroscopic sheath and a 0-degree telescope lens. It can be used to detect suture material, foreign matter, and lacerations of the urethra.

Management of Urethral Injury

Lacerations of the uethra should be repaired over a transurethral catheter in layers using No. 4-0 or 3-0 absorbable or delay-absorbable sutures. If the proximal urethra is involved, it is important to buttress the urethrovesical junction in an attempt to prevent the development of postoperative stress urinary incontinence. The use of a bulbocavernosus fat pad transplant should be considered if there is a need for additional tissue depth.

Postoperative genitourinary fistulas may leak urine immediately or after several weeks. Any loss of urine from the vagina should be evaluated promptly. If this examination suggests that the leakage is caused by a urethrovaginal, vesicovaginal, or ureterovaginal fistulal, it is important to perform endoscopy. In women with vesicovaginal or ureterovaginal fistula, it is important to perform endoscopy. In women with vesicovaginal or ureterovaginal fistulas, an intravenous urogram must be done to document the function of both renal units and to determine whether the fistula involves more than one organ. Posthysterectomy vesicovaginal fistulas are usually located just anterior to the vaginal cuff. On cystoscopy, they are usually located just above the interureteric ridge. Simple vesicovaginal fistulas that occur in the vaginal apex following an otherwise uncomplicated total hysterectomy are best treated by a partial apical colpocleisis.

BIBLIOGRAPHY

1. American College of Obstetricians and Gynecologists. Lower Urnary Tract Operative Injuries, ACOG Technical Bulletin 238. ACOG, Washington, DC, 1997.
2. Brubaker LT, Willbanks GD. Urinary tract injuries in pelvic surgery. Surg Lin North Am 1991;71:968.
3. Chan JK, Morrow J, Manetta A. Prevention of ureteral injuries in gynecologic. Logic surgery. Am J Obstet Gynecol 2003;188:1273.
4. Cruikshank SH. Surgical method of identifying the ureter during total Demel R. Ersatz des Ureters deurch eine Palstik aus der Harnblase (Vorlaufige Mitteilugg). Zentralbi Chir 1924;51:2008.
5. Giberti C, Germinale F, Lillo M, et al. Obstetric and gynaecological uretric injuries: Treatment and results, Br J Urol 1996;77:21.
6. Good No JA Jr. Powers TW, Harris VD. Ureteral injury in gynecologic surgery: A 10-year review in a community hospital. Am J Obstet Gynecol 1995;172:1817.
7. Hurt WG, Dunn Lj, (Eds). Complications of gynecologic surgery and trauma. In pincott, Pliladelphisa 1990.
8. Lee RA, Symmonds RE, Williams TJ. Current status of genito-urinary fistulas. Obstet Gynecol 1988;71:313.

9. Ostrzenski A, Radolinski B, Ostrzenska KM. A review of laparaoscopic ureteral injury in pelvic surgery. Obstet Gynecol Surv 2003;58:794.

10. Saidi MH, Sadler RK, Vancaillie TG, et al. Diagnosis and management of serious urinary complications after major operative laparoscopy. Obstet 1996;87:272.

CHAPTER 14

Dutta's New Approach for Abdominal TAH (Both Clamp and Clampless)

ABSTRACT

Abdominal hysterectomy is performed for various gynecological conditions. During operative procedures hemorrhage caused by trauma or slipping and retraction of uterine or ovarian artery has been a cause of great concern to gynecologists specially in absence of adequate blood transfusion facilities.

To overcome this problem, a new approach has been developed – ligation of the uterine artery and ovarian artery (in case of salpingo-ophorectomy) before going for conventional hysterectomy procedures.

500 cases of abdominal hysterectomy were performed during last 7 years. Traumatic injury to (L) uterine vessels was seen in 2(0.4%) cases. No other injury to ovarian vessels, (R) Uterine vessels, ureter and bladder were observed.

Hence, we conclude that ligation of uterine artery, prior to conventional abdominal hysterectomy procedures, is an extremely safe procedure reducing the risk of hemorrhage and thus allowing young gynecologists to perform this operation with less fear and more confidence.

In gynecological practice abdominal hysterectomy is performed in cases of dysfunctional uterine bleeding, fibroid uterus, endometriosis and cervical intraepithelial dysplasia, etc. Patients were usually suffering from moderate to severe anemia due to chronic blood loss in absence of proper treatment.

During operation hemorrhage caused by trauma or slipping and retraction of uterine artery or ovarian artery and injury to the ureter are great concern to the gynecologist specially at rural area where there is an inadequate blood transfusion facilities.

The author has undertaken a new approach to overcome such problem, i.e. during operation ligation of uterine and ovarian artery (in case of salpingo-oophorectomy) are performed prior to conventional hysterectomy procedures.

ANATOMY

It is important to know the anatomy of the uterine artery, ureter and bladder prior to abdominal hysterectomy procedures.

UTERINE ARTERY

It arises from anterior division of internal lilac artery. It passes through the base of broad ligament, where it deviates sharphy medially along with the uterine vein to cross over the ureter and then runs along the lateral border of uterus and to send collateral branches to the fundus where it forms a collateral anchor with the ovarian artery. It also gives off descending branches to cervix and vagina.

URETER (PELVIC PART)

About 1 cm above the ischial spine ureter turns inwards and forwards on the pelvic floor and in the base of the broad ligament, surrounded by veins of the vesical plexus and later by uterine veins, to the side of supravaginal cervix where it lies about 1.5 cm. from the cervix but rather closure on the left side than on the right. Here it is surrounded by uterine veins and passes under the uterine artery. After emerging from under the uterine artery, the ureter enters ureteric canal, formed in the pelvic connective tissues and then passes forwards and towards to the posterior wall of the bladder at the trigone.

BLADDER

The base of the bladder is closely related to the lower uterine segment and the anterior fornix of the vagina. The trigone of the bladder is continues with the upper one third of the vagina and anterior fornix, while the remainder of the bladder base rest intimately on the cervix and interior portion of lower uterine segment.

MATERIALS AND METHODS

These study were undertaken simultaneously at ESI Hospital, Cure Nursing Home, Kalyani and Greenview Nursing Home, Naihati, 24-Pgs (N) from January, 1987 to Oct. 1994. during these period 500 abdominal hysterectomy were performed by this procedure.

The patient was properly prepared for operation :

Operative Procedure (Clamp Hysterectomy)

1. After satisfactory general anesthesia, indwelling catheter is placed in the bladder for continuous drainage. A careful pelvic and rectovaginal examination were done first.
2. Abdomen is opened either by transverse or para-medium incision. Abdominal and pelvic cavity were evaluate properly to find out other concealed pathology.
3. Palpation of the lower portion of the pelvic ureter were done after exposing the pouch of Douglas.
4. The anterior leaf of broad ligament is incised from right to left round ligament. Wide mobilization and displacement of the bladder base from the cervix were done.

5. The posterior leaf of the broad ligament is incised down to the point where the ureterosacral ligament join the cervix.

6. Uterus was then pulled up by valsellum, two fingers were put posteriorly 1 cm. lateral from the uterine wall followed by lifting of the posterior broad ligament for exposing uterine artery. Uterine artery were completely skeletonized and exposed. Uterine antery were ligated by atraumatic 1-0 or by unab sorbable 1-0 suture – A_1 (primary step).

7. The same procedures were adopted in opposite side.

8. In case of salpingo-oophorectomy – (a) ligation of ovarian vessels along with infundibulopelvic ligament (B_1) by atraumatic 1-0 or any other suture were done first to be followed by (b) clamping, cutting and ligation of the ovarian vessels and infundibulopelvic ligament (B_2) which is to be proceeded by (c) clamping, cutting and ligation of the round ligament along with mesosalpinx (B_3) by transfixation suture (chromic-I) which ultimately passes beyond B_1 B_2 (Triple ligation). The same procedure were adopted in opposite side.

9. In case of total abdominal hysterectomy clamping, cutting and ligation of the (1) uterine end of the tube, mesosalpinge, ovarian branches of uterine artery, utero-ovarian ligament were performed.

10. Final step for clamping of uterine artery – Two clamp were applied – first one is placed at the level of the cervical os closed to the uterus. Second – placed at right angles to the lower uterine segment.

   The uterine vessels are cut with the scalpel between the First and Second clamp followed by freeing of uterine vessels from uterus by extending the incision around the tip of the 1st clamp – ligated by transfixation chromic catgut – 1 or 1-0 vickryl (A2) along with surrounding tissue of the uterine wall – to be followed by resulting the uterine vessels with surrounding tissue (A$_3$) (TRIPLE Ligation).

11. Same procedure were carried out in opposite site.
12. Mobilization of peritoneal flap from its attachment to the cervix up to posterior vaginal fornix were done.
13. Both uterosacral ligament clamped, incised and ligated with chromic catgut No. 1.
14. A plane between the cervix and vaginal wall anteriorly and anterior rectal wall and vagina posteriorly were made.
15. T-shaped incision is made in the fasia anterior to the cervix just below the level of the internal cervical os and ligated uterine vessels.
16. Clamping, cutting and ligating of cardinal ligament (both side) by chromic cat-gut-1 suture.
17. Opening of anterior vaginal fornix, cutting of posterior and lateral vaginal wall, removal of uterus along with the cervix, followed by closure of vagina by interrupted sutures by chromic-1-catgut.
18. Pelvic floor peritonized.
19. Abdomen is closed in layers.

Operative Procedure (Clampless Hysterectomy)

1. Same Procedure from Step 1 to 7
2. Ligation of infundibulopelvic ligament in case of salpingo-oophorectomy either one or both side or otherwise tying of fallopian tube, mesosalping, ovarian ligament to the uterus(both) in case of TAH.
3. Ligation of round ligament both side.
4. Second time ligation and incision of 2 and 3 in the same knot either in both side or one side depending upon the procedure.

5. Second time ligation and incision of uterine vessel on both side.
6. Identification, ligation and incision of (both) uterosacral ligament.
7. Identification, ligation and incision of cardinal ligament along with surrounding tissue.
8. Same procedure adopted in previous procedure 17 to 18.

OBSERVATION

Table 14.1: Indication for hysterectomy (n-500)

	Number	Percentage
Dysfunctional		
Uterine bleeding	275	55%
Fibroid uterus	170	34%
CIN III	20	4%
CIN II	5	1%
Endometriosis	20	4%
Carcinoma-in-situ	10	2%

Out 500 cases, 55% (275) had dysfunctional uterine bleeding, and 34% (170) had Fibroid uterus respectively. (Table 14.1).

Table 14.2: Type of operation (n-500)

	Number	Percentage
Total abdominal hysterectomy	60	12%
Total abdominal hysterectomy with (b) sided salpingo-oophorectomy	390	78%
Total abdominal hysterectomy with one sided salpingo-oophorectomy	50	10%

Total abdominal hysterectomy with both sided salpingo-oophorectomy were performed in most of the cases –78% (390) whereas 12% (20) cases had undergone total abdominal hysterectomy with one sided Salpingo-oophorectomy (Table 14.2).

Table 14.3: Operative complications (n-500)

	Number	Percent
Injury to (L) uterine vessels	2	4%
(R) uterine vessels	Nil	Nil
(R) ovarian vessels	Nil	Nil
(L) ovarian vessels	Nil	Nil
Urester	Nil	Nil
Bladder	Nil	Nil
Large intestine	Nil	Nil
Small intestine	Nil	Nil
Omentum	Nil	Nil

Injury to left uterine vessels were seen in 2 (0.4%) cases, has got statistically no significant (Table 14.3).

Table 14.4: Postoperative complication (n-500) (Within 10 days)

	Number	Percent
Primary healing	495	99%
Wound infection	5	1%
White discharge	3	0.6%
Bleeding per vagina	1	0.2%

495 (99%) had primary healing (Table 14.4).

Wound infection was in 5(1%) cases. Only 3(0.6%) had white discharge and 1(0.2%) had bleeding per vagina respectively.

It is observed from Table 14.5 that 5 (1%) had white discharge and 5 (1%) had low-back pain is found to be

Table 14.5: Follow-up upto – 1 year (in-410)

Wound	Healthy	—
Dyspareunia	Nil	—
Psychological	2	0.4%
White discharge	5	1%
Low backache	5	1%
Sexual problem	1	0.2%
Dysuria	2	0.4%

higher than of psychological 2(0.4%) and 1(0.2%) sexual problem, has got no statistical significance.

DISCUSSION

Abdominal hysterectomy is performed, for various gynecological condition. This type of patient had usually suffered from moderate to severe anemia due to chronic blood loss in absence of proper treatment.

In present gynecological practice, abdominal hysterectomy with or without salpingo-oophorectomy was done conventionally 1,2,3 from above downwards i.e. by clamping, cutting and ligating of the round ligament, uterine end of the tube, and utero-overian ligament, in-foundibulopelvic ligament followed by mobilization of bladder, exposing the uterine vessels for clamping, cutting and ligation, which is further followed by clamping, cutting and ligation of uterosacral, cardinal ligament, vaginal vault etc. respectively (both side).

During this procedure there may be traumatic injury to the vessels or slipping and retraction of uterine artery and ovarian artery especially in the hands of gynecologists (young). If it happens during operative procedure, there may be possibility of trauma to the ureter, bladder intestine and omentum, etc. due to inexperience of taking the emergency situation which is further aggravated by fear psychosis leading to unnecessary clamping in an unwanted area.

Hence to prevent such unwanted catastrophy a new approach i.e. ligation of uterine artery and ovarian artery (in case of salpingo-oophorectomy) were performed prior to conventional hysterectomy procedure as described in different standard surgery books 4,5.

It is very much important to know the anatomy of uterine artery and its course, pelvic ureter and bladder and lastly relationship between uterine artery and ureter, before proceeding such new technique.

During operative procedure – with retraction uterine corpus-ureters will usually fall 2 to 3 cm lateral and interior to the point of ligating uterine artery. Wide mobilization and displacement of bladder base from the cervix were done following separation of utero-vesical fold of peritoneum. The posterior lip of broad ligament incised, uterus is pulled up by valsellum, two figners were put posteriosly 1 cm above the uterine attachment of the uterosacral ligament and 1 cm lateral from the uterine wall followed by lifting of the perterior broad ligament for exposing the uterine artery. Uterine artery were completely skeletonized and exposed and ligated by atraumatic 1-0 with 30 mm needle or by unabsorbable 1-0 suture – A (Primary step).

Outmost care is to be taken while clamping the uterine arteries. First clamp is to be placed at the level of internal cervical os close to the uterus whereas second clamp placed at right angles to lower uterine segment to be followed by cutting of ligated (A_1) uterine vessels with the scalpel in between 1st and second clamp upto the tip of 1st clamp-ligated by transfixation suture (chromic catgut –1), or (vicryl 1-0) (A_2) along with the surrounding tissue of the uterine wall-which is to be followed by resuturing of A_1 and A_2 (A_3) (triple ligation).

It is also important to ligate the ovarian vessels along with infundibulopelvic ligament (B_1) by atraumatic 1-0 or vicryl (In case of salpingo-oophorectomy) to prevent slipping and retraction of ovarian vessels, which is to be followed by clamping, cutting and ligation of ovarian vessels along with infundibulopelvic ligament (B_2) by chromic –1 catgut. At last clamping, cutting and ligation of round ligament along with mesosalpinges (B_3) were done by transfixation suture (Chromic – 1) which is ultimately passes B_1 and B_2 (Tripple ligation).

Following this step-conventional hysterectomy procedures were advocated out-most care is to be taken while lightening of vaginal angle to secure proper hemostasis.

In present series, total abdominal hysterectomy with both sided salpingo-oophorectomy were performed in most of the cases – 78% (390) whereas 12% (60) cases had undergone total abdominal hysterectomy and 10% (50) cases had undergone total abdominal hysterectomy with one sided salpingo-oophoretomy.

In conventional hysterectomy procedures operative complications such as trauma or slipping and retraction of uterine artery and ovarian artery leading to hematoma is very much significant as reported by various author is 6, 7, 8 in time to time. There may be also injury to ureter 9, 10, 11 bladder intestine and omentum etc. which was usually happened while tackling hematoma and hemorrhagic situation during operative procedures.

In present series no traumatic injury to right uterine vessels, left and right ovarian vessels, ureter and bladder omentum and intestine were reported except 2 (0.4%) had traumatic injury to (L) uterine vessels which was managed immediately, has got statistically no significance.

The disadvantage following this operation were (1) Occasionally there may be traumatic injury to uterine and ovarian vessels (2) anatomical variation of uterine or ovarian or aberrant artery and ureter may cause problem (but not seen in this series – 3). Broad ligament fibroid, endometriosis, severe adhesion and fixed uterus may cause operative problem which can be managed first by adopting conventional procedure till the region of uterine artery reached where uterine artery was properly exposed, skeletonized and ligated to prevent slipping and retraction of uterine artery prior to traditional clamping of uterine vessels. (4) lastly accidental ligation of ureter if happens may sometimes cause problem.

Main advantages of this operation were

1. No slipping and retraction of uterine and ovarian artery.
2. Minimum blood loss.
3. Avoidance of unnecessary clamping while tackling hematoma and hemorrhagic situation.
4. Avoidance of ureter, bladder and intestinal injury.
5. Good and safe for young gynecologist.
6. Better recovery.

Hence we conclude that ligation of uterine artery prior to conventional abdominal hysterectomy is extremely safe procedures, reducing the risk of hemorrhage, and thus allowing young gynecologists to perform this operation with less fear and more confidence.

COMMENTS

Prof Hanslin Demann (Germany) - 4.12.93

In my opinion this recommended technique is a good one for teaching beginners

Prof Adam Ostrzenki (USA) – 4.12.93
This is a way to go

Prof Minoo Chinoy (USA) – 4.12.93
This technique is good for teaching

Prof Jordon Philips (verbal)
This is a good approach

This paper presented at
1. Video-demonstration- XXXVIII All India Obstt. Gynaecological Conf. Elliot hall, NRS Medical college, Calcutta, WB – dec 27–30, 1993.
2. Video-demonstration-All India NAVSRWI Conf, JIPMAR, Pondicherry - sept, 1994.
3. Video-demonstration-AICOG, Bangalore, 1998
4. Video-demonstration-FIGO world congress Denmark – 1997
5. Video-demonstration-FIGO world congress Washinton – 2000
6. Video-demonstration-FIGO world congress Chile, - 2003, Kuwalampur-2006
7. Live-demonstration-AICOG, Agra, -2004.

REFERENCES

1. Richardson. A simplified technic for abdominal panhysterectomy surg. Gynaecol Obstet 1929;48-428.
2. Dicker RCI, Scally MJ, Greenspan JR, et al. Hysterectomy among women of reproductive age: Trends in the United States JAMA, 1982;248-323:1970-8.
3. Richard F, Mattingly Jhon, Thompson D. Telinde's Operative Gyanegology, sixth edition, chapter 2, 1989;203-55.
4. Jhon Howkins, Sir John Stall Worthy. Bonney's Gynaecological Surgery, eight edition, chapter 14, 298-313.

5. Howard W. Jones III, Anne Colston Weniz, Ionnie S. Burnet. "Novak's Textbook of Gynaecology" "Abdominal Hysterectomy" 11th edition, 1988;29-32.

6. Gram LA. Open cuff method of abdominal hysterectomy obstet, Gynecol 1975;46:42.

7. Robinson N RE. Abdominal hysterectomy: Total and sub total, Operative Surgery, Chares Rob, Rodney Smith (Eds): 3rd edition, 169-71,1976-1978.

8. Miyazawa K. Technique for total abdominal hysterectomy: Historical and Clinical Perspective, Obstet, Gynaecol Surv 1992;47(7):433-47 (100 ref).

9. Kamala Jayaram VV. J Obstet and Gynec of India, 1992;42(6):8336-9.

10. More JC. J Obstet and Gynec. Brit C 'Wealth' 1973;80:508.

11. Russel Matinak LMD, Carola Wheeler, MD. Therapeutic Gynecologic Procedure—Current Obstetric and Gynaecologic Diagnosis and Treatement. Alam H Decherney, Martin L (Eds): Pernou, 8th 1994;884-905.

CHAPTER 15

Descent Vaginal Hysterectomy (DVH) [Ward Mayo's]

WARD MAYO'S OPERATION

Vaginal hysterectomy plus pelvic floor repair (PFR) done under general or spinal anesthesia.

Indications

1. Any degree uterine prolapse where uterus is diseased.
2. Any degree uterine prolapse with normal uterus.
3. Postmenopausal woman.

Contraindication

    I. Repair of VVF RVF
   II. Pelvic endometrosis
  III. Severe adhesion
  IV. Big ovary – An tumour
   V. 20wk fibroid
  VI. Post radiation vagina
 VII. Narrow vagina.

Steps

1. Routine preliminary preparation for the vaginal operation is done.
2. Incision is made on vaginal attachment cervix.
3. The steps of anterior colporrhaphy are followed till the bladder is pushed up and the uterovesical pouch of peritoneum is exposed. The latter pouch is opened by a transverse incision (anterior colpotomy). A narrow bladed 'L' shaped retractor (Landon's bladder retractor) is introduced through the anterior colpotomy opening to retract the bladder behind the symphysis pubis.
4. Posterior colpotomy (opening of the pouch of Douglas) is done through the incision on the posterior cervicovaginal junction.

5. The uterus is eventrated (fundus is brought out) through the anterior colpotomy opening by hooking the fundus by a finger or the volsellum or cat's paw. The fundus is pulled by the volsellum after bringing out.

6. The uterus is severed form its lateral attachments by three pairs of clamps placed on each side as close to the uterus as possible from below upwards as follows. Thus vaginal hysterectomy is done.

   a. **First pair** is placed one on each side to include the cardinal and uterosacral ligaments (clamps are applied from below and these structures are divided between the clamp and the cervix). These pedicles are tied by chromic catgut replacing clamps on either side.

   b. **Second pair** is placed to include uterine vessels on each side and the latter are divided between the clamp and uterus. Pedicle is tied on either side.

   c. **Third pairs** to include fallopian tube, ligament of the ovary, round ligament, mesosalpinx. These structures are divided in between clamp and fundus. Pedicle is tied by chromic catgut on either side.

7. The ends of ligated predicted on each side are tied in the midline with that of the corresponding pedicles **except the pedicle for uterine vessels**. The pelvic peritoneum is closed by catgut ligature before the approximation of the pedicles.

8. In case of enterocele, posteriorly the pounch of Douglas is dissected, excised after securing the base by a ligature. Below this, the uterosacral ligaments are sutured in the midline with catgut sutures. This repair of enterocele is done before approximation of the broad ligament pedicles. The approximate pedicle

of uterosacral and Mackenrodt ligaments are fixed to the posterior vaginal vault by a transfixation suture.

9. anteriorly, the bladder is supported by midline suturing of the vesicle fascia as in anterior colporrhaphy. At the depth, bladder fascia is fixed to the uppermost broad ligament pedicles (ovarian ligament, tube and round ligament) so that, hiatus between the bladder and broad ligaments is closed.

10. Redundant portions of the vaginal flaps are excised and the wound is approximated by interrupted catgut 0 sutures.

11. Posterior colpoperineorrhaphy is performed to narrow the dilated vagina and its introitus.

CHAPTER 16

Nondescent Vaginal Hysterectomy (NDVH)

Cervix cannot be pulled to vaginal introitus as in uterine prolapse but inside vagina below the level of ischial spine. Mobility of uterus is most important factor in NDVH.

Indications

1. DUB,
2. Uterine fibroid–pelvic size,
3. Adenomyosis,
4. CIN,
5. Cervical and adenometrial polyp.

Contraindications

1. Uterus larger that 16 weeks,
2. Narrow vagina,
3. VVF repaired,
4. Extensive pelvic endometriosis.

STEP OF OPERATION IN CASE OF DUB

1. Anesthesia – general or spinal, lithotomy position with buttocks at edge of the table. Preoperative cephalosporin antibiotic is given.
2. Circumferential incision is made on vaginal attachments to cervix.
3. Dissection of posterior vaginal flap till Douglas pouch opened. Blade of sim's speculum is inserted into Douglas pouch.
4. Smaller sim's speculum retracts anterior vaginal flap for dissection of bladder till uterovesical pouch is opened through which sim's speculum blade is inserted to retract the bladder.
5. **First pair of clamps** is applied on uterosacral ligament, cut between clamp and cervix. All divided

pedicles except uterine arteries are tied by vicryl suture on both sides.

6. By second pair, Mackenrodt ligament is clamped, cut between clamp and cervix.

7. By third pair, uterine arteries are clamped, cut between clamp and cervix one on either side and ligated.

8. Fundus is now delivered through Douglas pouch, fundal attachments on either side are clamped, cut between clamp and fundus, thus uterus is removed.

   If adnexa is removed, fundal clamp is placed on infundibulopelvic ligament cut and ligated.

9. Peritoneum is closed by pursestring catgut suture.

10. Fundal and paracervical pedicles are tied to each other in midline (this is simplified by author).

11. Vagina is closed transversely using a continuous catgut suture.

12. Vagina is packed with betadine soaked roller gauze and removed after 24 hours.

13. Self retaining Foley catheter is kept for 48 hours.

CONCLUSION

For indications where both abdominal and vaginal hysterectomy can be performed. NDVH is the best.

Complications

   I. Hemorrhage – broad ligament hematoma – due to slipping of uterine vessels/ovarian vessles.

  II. Injury to ureter in case prolonged prolapse in old women, preview operative scar on uterus.

 III. Intraperitoneal hemorrhage

  IV. Injury to rectum, bladder and urethra – (VVF, RVF)

   V. Vaginal scar.

CHAPTER 17

Vaginal Hysterectomy for Difficult Cases

BIG UTERUS

Uterus above 14 week size is very difficult to remove per vagina. In case if it is to be removed after separating the bladder and rectum carefully and opening the pouch of Douglas and anterior iterovesical pouch , cervix is hold by tissue forcep(2) and pulled downwards . Uterus is bisected .Clamping of all the pedicules from above downwards will be done first (which side is easier) to be followed by other side.

FIBROID UTERUS

Uterus above 14 week size is very difficult to remove per vagina. In case if it is to be removed after separating the bladder and rectum carefully and opening the pouch of Douglas and anterior uterovesical pouch , cervix is hold by tissue forcep(2) and pulled downwards . Uterus is bisected or opening. After opening the uterus submucous fibroid or interstitial fibroid either single or double can be removed first (myomectomy) to be followed by removal of the uterus by clamping of all the pedicules from above downwards will be done first (which side is easier) to be followed by other side. In case of subserous fibroid morcellation of fibroid will be done first before applying the clamp on the cornue. In case of cervical fibroid the myomectomy should be done first to be followed by hysterectomy.

SEVERE ADHESION

Care should be taken not to injure the ureter, bladder, urethra and rectum while dissecting the structures.

CHAPTER 18

Complication and Management Following Vaginal Hysterectomy Operation

DURING OPERATION

Hemorrhage and Hematoma

Prevention

1. Ligation of uterine artery prior to VH procedure (Dutta' technique)
2. Proper dissection of bladder and urethra in suspected addition of bladder and urethra to the uterus. Ana adnexa
3. Proper hemostat before closing any wound.
4. Ligation of infundibulopelvic ligament before removal of ovary.

Curative

1. Immediate blood transfusion.
2. Proper hemostatis measures in locally detected bleeding.
3. If intra-abdominal bleeding immediate laparotomy or laparoscopy.
4. Ligation of internal iliac artery or uterine artery.
5. Vault bleeding by secondary suture.

Injury to the Bladder, Urethra and Ureter

Prevention

1. Proper dissection of bladder and urethral in case of adhesion to the uterus.
2. Care to the taken
3. Injury to the anus and rectum to locate the site of ureter in long standing prolapse or any adhesions in pouch of Douglas

Curative

1. Immediate repair of bladder in 3 layers by absorbable suture.

2. Uerthral injury repaired with absorbable suture.
3. Indwelling catheter for 21 days .
4. For ureteral injury –Laparotomy –Identification of injure site and immediate repair.
5. Assistant from uro-surgeon is mandatory.

Injury to the Anus and Rectum

1. Identification and repair in three layers by absorbable suture
2. Postoperative bowel care
3. Antibiotic

Vault Hematoma and Infection

Drainage, antibiotic and blood transfusion.

Maternal Mortality and Morbidity

Good operative technique and care no maternal mortality reporated but morbidity can be reduced by adopting good nutrition ,prevention of anemia ,maintenance of hygiene.

CHAPTER 19

Dutta's New Approach for Vaginal Hysterectomy (Clampless)

Dutta's Clampless (five step) operation for descent and non-descent vaginal hysterectomy (200 cases)

First Step

Dissection of anterior vaginal flap and bladder wall till uterovesical pouch is opened. Dissection of posterior vaginal flap till Douglas pouch is opened.

Second Step

Ligation of uterine artery (B) is done, by putting 2 finger (in the pouch of Douglas) 1 cm above and 1 cm lateral to the insertion of uterosacral attachment of the uterus, (by catgut or vicryl +-0). Care to be taken not to injure the ureters rectum, etc.

Third Step

Uterosacral ligament (B), is identified tied by vicryl 1-0, t Mackerdrodt ligament is identify, tied by vicryl 1-0, then cut.

Fourth Step

Uterine arteries (B) along with lateral uterine structure is ligated, tied and then cut.

Fifth Step

Fundus is now delivered through uterovesical pouch – (1) if adnexa removed – ligation of infundibulopelvic ligament (twice) by vicryl (1-0) and them cut. (2) if adnexa not removed – funded attachment of fallopian tube, utero-ovarian ligament, round ligament along with mesosalping are ligated by vicryl (1-0,) and then cut (viii) others method as performed in ward mayos operation.

Advantages

1. No slipping of uterine and ovarian arteries.
2. Less vaginal trauma.
3. More space for operative field (occupied by Instrument).
4. No injury toureter, bladder.
5. Loss of blood less.
6. Good recovery.

Disadvantage

1. Big uterus – 14 weeks size
2. Severe adhesion
3. Endometriosis.

Complication

1. Injury to uterine vessels (L) = 1%
2. Injury to uterine vessels (R) = 5%
3. Slipping of uterosacral ligament = 0.1%.

CHAPTER 20

Documentation for Hysterectomy Operation Case

SECTION I

- Monthly Serial Number
- Yearly Serial Number
- Name and Address.
- Age, Parity, Religion.
- Past History of any disease.

SECTION II

- Record of all investigation report.
- Record of advantage note.
- Record of preoperative note.
- Record of all preoperative findings.
- Provisional diagnosis.
- Date of admission
- Informed consent.
- Preoperative drug use.

SECTION III

- Date of operation
- Record of drug used including anesthetic drug.
- Palce of operation.
- Types of operation – AH /VH.
- Details operation note, including anesthetic note.
- Video recording in selected cases.
- Name of team of Doctor.
- Note of vault closure by CAT / VICRYL
- Macroscopic evaluation of operated specimen.
- Operative diagnosis.

SECTION IV

- Histopathological examination of whole specimen.
- Final diagnosis to be informed to the patient.
- Next visit to the informed or before that if any complication.
- Record of HRT drug and follow-up if prescribed.
- Postoperative drug to be recorded.
- Follow up to 1 year.

All women undergoing hysterectomy in my case were counceled property regarding the advantages and disadvantages of removal of ovary during hysterectomy and also explained the menopausal problem if any after hysterectomy.

Regarding removal of ovary or not authors adopted and maintained following principle. There are (i) < 40 yr = Both ovary intact (except premature menopause due to PMOF and ovarian cancer). (ii) 40 – 45 yr = (B) ovary intact (except I + Ovarian endometriosis + TO Mass + Ovarian abscess) (iii) 45-48 yr = One ovary intact (iv) > 48 yr = Removal of (B) ovary.

All ovary should be subjected for HPE.

CHAPTER 21

Epidemiological Survey— Hysterectomy for Fibroid Uterus

Total hysterectomy	5000
Period of operation (1990-2005)	15 years

Abdominal hysterectomy	3220
Vaginal hysterectomy	1550
Subtotal hysterectomy	135
Cesarean hyterectomy	595

A. Abdominal hysterectomy (no-3220)

TAH	1750
TAH one sided salpingo-oophorectomy	875
TAH and BSO	595

A1. Indication (no- 3220)

DUB	915
Fibroid	1780
Adenomyosis	72
Endometriosis	20
TO mass	75
Dysplasia	46
CIN-I	32
CIN-II	20
Ovarian tumor	240
Others	20

A2. Place of fibroid (n –1780)

Uterus (N-1550)	Interstitial fibroid 1250
	Submucous 270
	Subserous 30
Cervix (N- 134)	Anterior 52
	Posterior 36
	Lateral 34
	Central 12

Broad ligament	True 56
(N-96)	False 40

A3. Number of fibrod(no-1780)

1.	350
2–4	990
4-6	310
Above 6-130	

A4. Symptoms

Symptoms	MH			Pain abdomen		Lump abdomen	UTI problem	Vowel problem
	R	I	E	No	Yes			
Inter-stitial (1250)	59%	25%	18%	69%	31%	33%	29%	11%
Sub-mucous (270)	2%	4%	96%	35%	65%	12%	9%	2%
Subserous (30)	93%	51%	2%	76%	24%	27%	2%	11%
Cervical (134)	92%	6%	2%	14%	86%	39%	65%	59%
Broad ligament (96)	89%	9%	2%	13%	87%	11.5%	2.5%	7%

MH—Menstrual history
R—Regular
I—Irregular
E—Excessive

A5. Associated macroscopic findings

Ovarian cyst	(R) 172
	(L) 129
	(B) 205
TO mass	517
Chocolate cyst	252

Endometriosis	736
Dermoid cyst	60
PID	207
Tuberculosis	16

A.6

a. HPE of fibriod (n=1780)

Leiomyoma	1562
With adenomyosis	102
Hyaline degeneration	49
Cystic degeneration	28
Red degeneration	3
Necrosis of myoma	15
Calcified cyst	26
Leiomyosarcoma	7

b. HPE of cervix, endometrium, ovary and fallopian tube (n=1780)

A. Cervix

Cervicitis	1496
Dysplasia	145
Hyperplasia	52
Cin i	36
Cin ii	29
Carcinoma *in situ*	17
Ca-cervix(invasive)	5

B. Endometrium

Secretory	1582
Hyperplasia no atypia	119
Hyperplasia with atypia	75
Ca endometrium	4

C. Ovary

Follicular cyst	1240
Corpus luteum cyst	291
Mucinous cyst	189

	Serous cyst	17
	Brenner tumor	3
	Dermoid cyst	10
	Ovarian endometriosis	20
	Serous cystadenocarcinoma	1
	Others	9
D.	Fallopian tube	
	Normal	1350
	Salpingitis	430

Age (no: 1780)

< 30 years	105
30-35 years	329
35-40 years	851
40-45 years	255
45-50 years	162
50-60 years	46
> 60 years	32

Parity

Nulliparous	310
1	815
2-3	475
4-5	105
Above 5	75

Socioeconomic status

Poor	920
Average	771
Good	89

Religion

Hindu	177
Muslim	700
Sikh	nil
Others	3

CONCLUSION

Following observation were seen from this survey that fibroid is found

1. To be more in advancing age
2. Poor socioeconomic status patients
3. Ovarian cyst most predominently associted with
4. Significant pathological changes in endometrium, cervix, overy.
5. Branners tumor is seen in postmenopausal women suffering from fibroid.

CHAPTER 22

Postmenopausal Care and Hormone Replacement Therapy

POSTOPERATIVE ADVISE (POA)

Walking after 1 month (in obese and diabetic patient) of surgery.

Exercise after 2 month (in all cases) of surgery

Diet contain fruit juice and fat free low calorie diet.

Sexual activity after 2 month.

WHY POSTOPERATIVE ADVISE ?

- To reduce weight.
- To control diabetes and hypertension.
- To prevent cardiovascular disease, osteopenia, osteoporosis.
- To control-age related muscular dystrophy
- Early detection and recognization of menopausal syndrome.

POSTOPERATIVE CHECK-UP

- Visit – 6 wk, 1, 2, 3, months and 1 year.
- Search for – Vasomotor symptoms, mental status, sexual status.
- Check for– Weight, hypertension, cardiovascular system, breast, any bone tenderness.
- Look for – Muscle wasting/obesity/gynecological pathology, etc.
- Investigation for–(Every visit) Lipid profile, sugar, ECG stool examination.
- Sent for – Hormone profile – FHS, LH, estradiol after 3 months, 6 months and 1 year of surgery.
- Screen for – Osteoporosis/osteopenia by dosimetry (in case of previous history of estrogen deficiency osteopenia or osteoporosis, drug induced osteoporosis, and diabetic).

HRT FOR POST HYSTERECTOMY CASES

Total No. cases—5000

Level I Care—Reduction of body weight by walking and exercise, low calori fat free diet and calcium tab are prescribed for all women .

Good respond 4372 case within one year

Poor respond 628

Level II Care—With vasomotor symptoms - level I care plus isoflavin

Total no of cases –325

Good respond –25

Poor respond -300

With history of estrogen deficiency or osteopenia - Level I care plus estrogen replacement therapy (Premarin, Progynova)

Total no of cases –303

Good respond –100

Poor respond –203

Level III Care

Level I care plus

i. Failed estrogen hormone replacement therapy (no 203),

ii. Failed isoflavain treament (300)

iii. Cases of osteopenia and early osteoporosis (11)

iv. Past history of irregular period –(4)

v. Past history of cardiovascular disease (7)

vi. Premature menopause (3)

TIBOLONE (LIVIAL TAB) [ORGANON]

Dose- 1 tab daily for 28 days x 6 cycle

Monitoring as per postoperative check up
Respond 612 not respond 16 (drug taken irregularly).

ADVANTAGE OF TAKING TIBOLONE (LIVIAL)

- Relieve hot flushes, night sweats,
- Elevates mood
- Improves libido and sex life
- Prevents urogenital problems
- Protection from osteoporosis and fractures
- Protection from heart attacks and strokes
- No periods
- Safe over long-term use.

FACTS ABOUT MENOPAUSE AND HRT

Menopause is defined as the permanent cessation of menstruation resulting from the loss of ovarian activity.
Menopause

Natural   Artificial
                                 Surgical   Radiation

Median age of menopause
In western
Countries   : 50 + years

In India   : 40 years
Population of postmenopausal women in India
Population aged 50 years

Premenopause
- Fertile period
- Regular cycles

MENOPAUSE OCCURS

After about 35 years of regular periods, ovary runs out of the supply of eggs and fails to respond to commands from headquater.

Hormone production gets reduced

No more
Pregnancy   Aging process
                                          starts affecting all
No more mense   parts of the body

Symptoms of Menopause

Early Symptoms

- Perimenopausal menstrual changes
- Vasomotor instability :
  Hot flushes, night sweats, vertigo, palpitation and weakness.

Intermediate Symptoms

- Atrophic changes:
  vagina, urinary tract, breast, skin
- Psychological changes:
  Irritability, depression, anxiety.
  Insomnia, crying spells, loss of libido, loss of self confidence.

Psychological Symptoms

- Anxiety and fear
- Depression and irritability
- Lethargy and insomnia
- Loss of concentration and forgetfulness
- Loss of libido
- Somatic symptoms

More than 50% of postmenopausal women suffer from urogenital problems

Relative frequency of climateric symptoms

Symptoms

Hot Flushes

Urinary complaints

Vaginal complaints

Joint / muscle pain

Psychological

Insomnia.

Long term complications

- Osteoporosis
- Cardiovascular disease
  Heart attack, stroke
- Alzheimer's disease.

PATTERN OF BONE LOSS WITH AGE

Peak bone density

RISK FACTORS FOR DEVELOPMENT OF OSTEOPOROSIS

- Female sex
- Loss of ovarian function
- Race – European or Asian
- Poor diet in childhood
- Excessive alcohol India
- Low calcium intake
- Low body weight
- Nulliparity
- Heavy smoking
- Less exercise

Prevention of osteoporosis is possible if
- Diet is rich in calcium and diary products.
- Exposure to sun light is sufficient
- Exercises are done regularly
- Smoking and alchohol is avoided.

OSTEOPOROSIS AND HRT

Prevention of Osteoporosis

- Maximum benefits if HRT is initiated at the onset of menopause
- HRT prevents bone loss in all stages of post-menopausal life
- HRT for 5 years reduces lifetime incidence of fracture of the femur by approximately 50%.

CARDIOVASCULAR DISEASE

Increased incidence of arterial disease in postmenopause is due to

$\uparrow$ Bad cholesterol LDL - C

$\downarrow$ Good cholesterol HDL - C

Annual incidence of cardiovascular disease per 1000 women

Age

CARDIOVASCULAR DISEASE AND HRT

- HRT reduction of coronary heart disease risk
- Postmenopausal estrogen use leads to a reduction of the relative risk of coronary heart disease (CHD)
- 35% reduction of CHD risk has been found in past and current HRT – users in comparison to never – users, this effect is more pronounced in current than in past - users

HRT

Menopause is a hormone deficient state and HRT replaces these hormones from outside.

It contains estrogen/progestogen/androgen.

- Estrogen: Ideal hormone as menopause is an estrogen deficient state.
- Progestogen: Reduces the risk of uterine. Cancer caused by estrogen.
- Androgen: Takes care of mood libido

BENEFITS OF HRT

Short-term benefits for
- Hot flushes, night sweats
- Genito urinary problems
- Psychological problems

COMMON HRT AVAILABLE IN INDIA

Oral

Evalon/evalon forte tablets, premarin tablets, progynova tablets.

Transdermal

Estraderm patch, system patch, sandrenal ge.

Vaginal Cream

Evalon cream, vagifem cream.

Hormone replacement therapy

New trends

A NEW APPROACH TO HRT (TIBOLONE)

- Relieve hot flushes, night sweats,
- Elevates mood
- Improves libido and sex life
- Prevents urogenital problems
- Protection from osteoporosis and fractures
- Protection from heart attacks and strokes
- No periods
- Safe over long-term use.

MYTH VS REALITY CURRENT AWARENESS

- Low level of awareness
- Suspicious of hormones and HRT
- Know and use only for short-term symptoms
- Confused by conflicting feedback from different gynecologists
- Feel HRT is irrelevant Indian scenario.

HRT AND CANCER

- Cancer of uterus: risk is nil with additional progestogen therapy. and no risk with tibolone.
- Cancer of breast; Almost no risk if HRT is given or < 9 years

Contraindications

- Undiagnosed vaginal bleedings:
- Suspected or known estrogen depending tumor;
- Active/severe liver disease.

PRE-TREATMENT ASSESSMENT

History

- Symptoms of estrogen deficiency.
- H/o DVT, liver disease, estrogen dependent tumor etc.
- H/o operation for removal of estrogen dependent tumor.
- Family history of breast cancer, IHD/CVA, osteoporosis in (1st degree relative)
- H/o previous therapy with hormone.

Common Side Effects of HRT

- Due to estrogen
- Leg cramps
- Breast tenderness
- Fluid retention
- Weight gain
- Nausea
- Vaginal discharge
- Due to progestogen
- Abdominal cramps
- Backache
- Fluid retention
- Weight gain
- Breast tenderness
- Depressed mood and inability.

Physical Examination

- Body weight
- BP
- Breast examination,
- Pelvic examination

Investigations

- Vaginal/cervical (pap) smear
- TV sonography
- Endometrial sampling
- Memmography
- Liver function test
- PPBS

Follow-up Visits

- Enquiry about improvement of symptoms, side : effects and vaginal bleeding.
- Checking body weight blood pressure 6 monthly.
- Cervical/vaginal smear yearly.
- Remammography 2/3/5 yearly.
- LFT. PPBS yearly.

CHAPTER 23

Color Photo of Hysterectomy Cases

Figures 23.1 to 23.37 show various causes, techniques and procedures of abdominal hysterectomy and update modifications made therein.

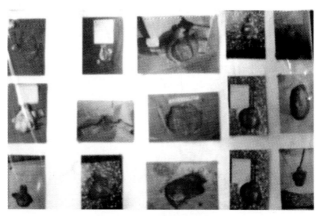

Fig. 23.1: Types of fibroid

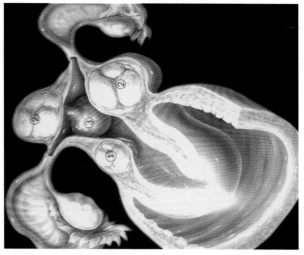

Fig. 23.2: Different types of fibroid uterus

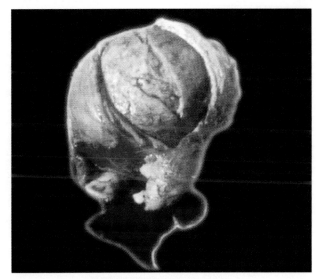

Fig. 23.3: Submucous fibroid

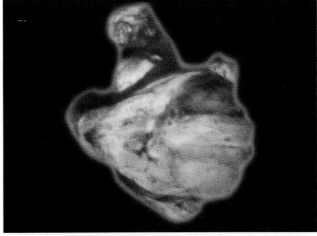

Fig. 23.4: Submucous fibroid

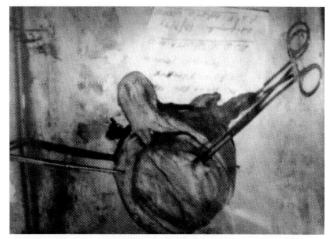

Fig. 23.5: Submucous fibroid

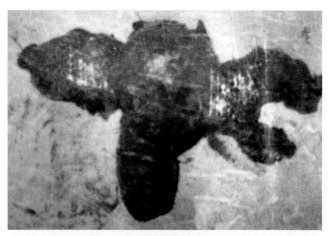

Fig. 23.6: Fibroid with TO mass

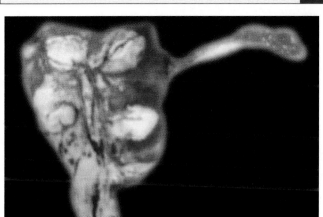

Fig. 23.7: Multiple fibroid

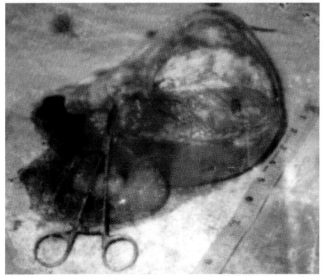

Fig. 23.8: Interstitial fibroid with fetus

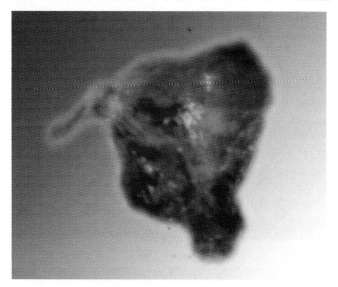

Fig. 23.9: Broad ligament fibroid (true)

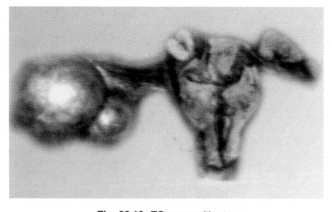

Fig. 23.10: TO mass with uterus

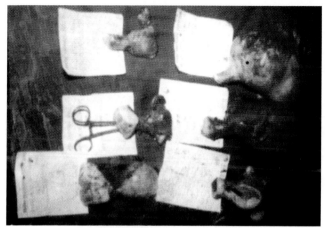

Fig. 23.11: Picture of DUB and fibroid

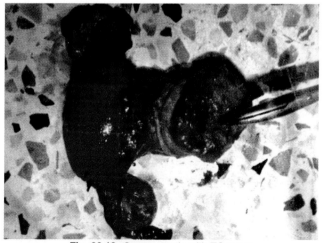

Fig. 23.12: Cancer cervix with TO mass

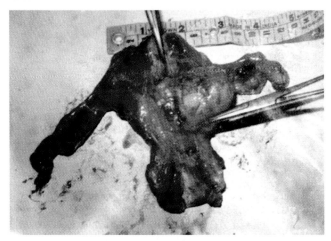

Fig. 23.13: Endometrial cancer with TO mass

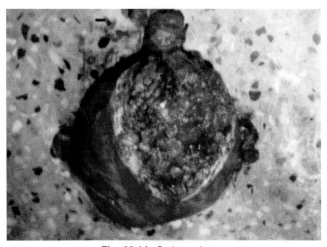

Fig. 23.14: Coriocarcinoma

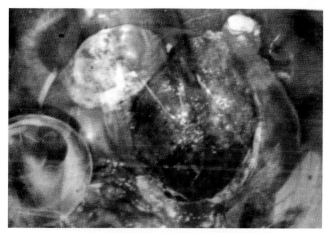

Fig. 23.15: Endometrial cancer with ovarian cancer

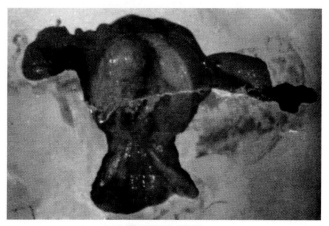

Fig. 23.16: DUB

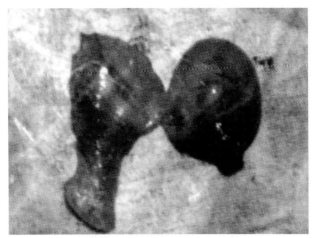

Fig. 23.17: Left ovarian cyst

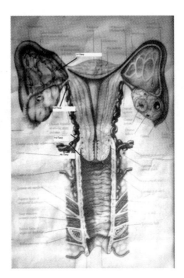

Fig. 23.18: Original Ridhardson's procedure
for abdominal hysterectomy

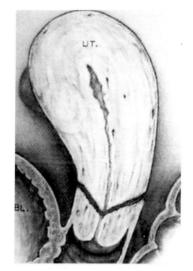

Fig. 23.19: Steps of subtotal hysterectomy

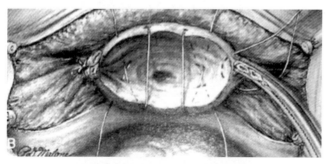

Fig. 23.20: Closure of cervical wound following removal of the uterus (subtotal hysterectomy) by Vicryl-1-0

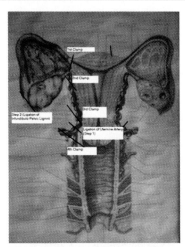

Fig. 23.21: Dutta's new approach of abdominal
hysterectomy (clamp) before 1995

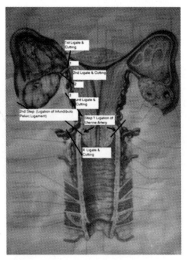

Fig. 23.22: Dutta's new approach of abdominal
hysterectomy (clampless) after 1995

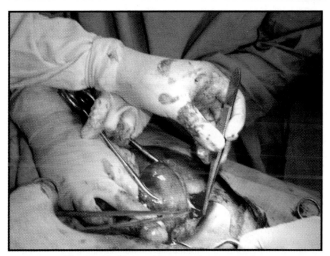

Fig. 23.23: Steps of hysterectomy operation

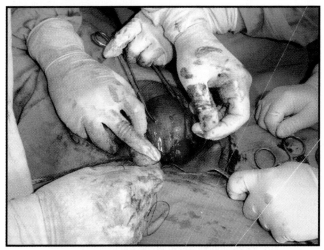

Fig. 23.24: Ligation of uterine artery

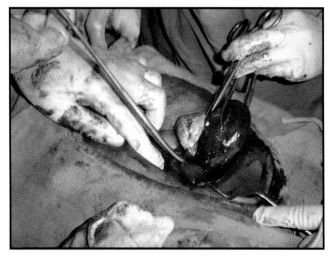

Fig. 23.25: Ligation of infundibulo pelvic ligament

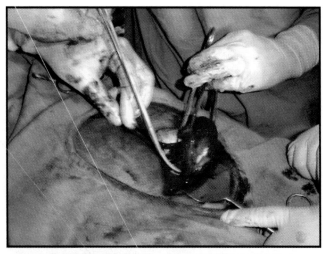

Fig. 23.26: Identification of the round ligament and
then ligate, tying and cutting

VAGINAL HYSTERECTOMY OPERATION

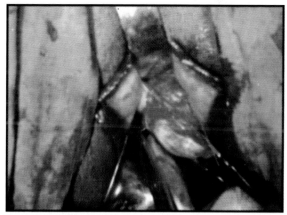

Fig. 23.27: Ligature passed through right uterosacral ligament

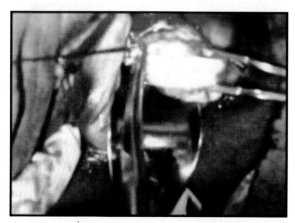

Fig. 23.28: Traction on right uterosacral ligament before cutting

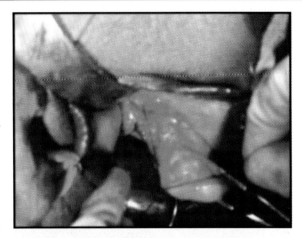

Fig. 23.29: Ligating the right uterine vessels

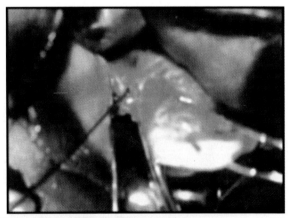

Fig. 23.30: The right uterine vessels being cut after doubly tying

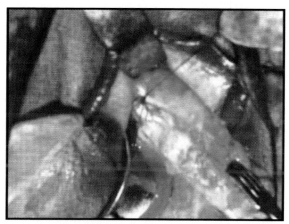

Fig. 23.31: Ligating the lower part of the broad ligament

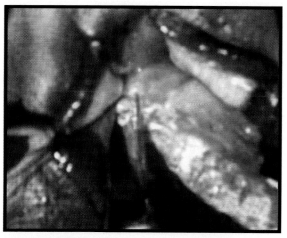

Fig. 23.32: Applying traction on and cutting
the lower part of right broad ligament

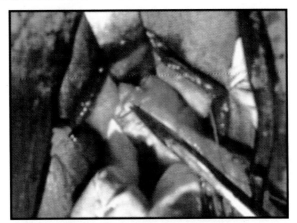

Fig. 23.33: Finger hooked behind ovarian and round ligament and first ligature taken

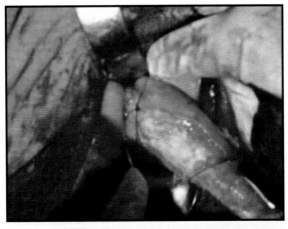

Fig. 23.34: Right ovarian and round ligament being tied

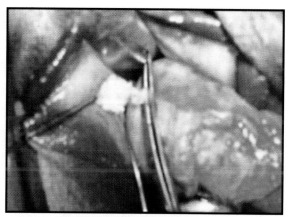

Fig. 23.35: Right fundal structures cut

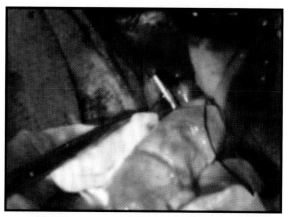

Fig. 23.36: A straight artery forceps behind fundal
structures for taking free tie

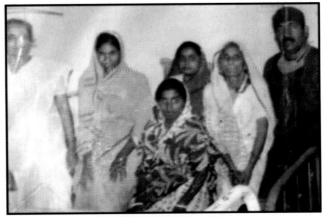

Fig. 23.37: Doctor with patients

CHAPTER 24

Complication of Hysterectomy— A Comparative Analysis

Table 24.1: Complication of hysterectomy—A comparative analysis

Complication	Other series Abdominal	Other series Vaginal	LAVH	Dutta's series Abdominal	Dutta's series Vaginal
Bleeding					
Hemorrhage	1-2%	1-5%	1%	0.5%	0.2%
Transfusion	2-12%	2-8.3%	1.58%	1%	0.1%
Injuries					
Bladder	1-2%	0.5-1.5%	1%	0.05%	0.01%
Ureter	0.1-0.5%	0.05-0.1%	0.19%	Nil	Nil
Bowel	0.1-1%	0.1-0.8%	0.1-1%	0.05%	Nil
Vesicovaginal fistula	0.1-0.2%	0.1-0.2%	0.22%	Nil	Nil
Pelvic infection	3.2-10%	3.9-10%	1.27%	2.7-5%	3.5-10.3%
UTI	1.1-5%	1.7-5%	0.81%	6.2-8.5%	5.3-8.9%
Vault					
Bleeding	—	—	—	1.2%	2.2%
Prolapse	—	—	—	0.01%	0.02%
Sexual				Good	Good
HRT				2.2%	Nil

Source:
John A Rock, et al. Te Linde's Operative Gynecology. 9th edn 2003;824.
Dutta et al. New Approach of Abdominal Hysterectomy, 1995-2005.

INDEX